W9-BZM-118

Making Health Reform Work

Making Health Reform Work

THE VIEW FROM THE STATES

John J. DiIulio, Jr.
Richard R. Nathan
editors

The Brookings Institution
Washington, D.C.

Copyright © 1994
THE BROOKINGS INSTITUTION
1775 Massachusetts Avenue, N.W., Washington, D.C. 20036

All rights reserved

Library of Congress Cataloging-in-Publication data:

Making health reform work : the view from the states / John J.
   DiIulio, Jr., Richard R. Nathan, editors.
       p.   cm.
   Includes bibliographical references and index.
   ISBN 0-8157-1852-7 (cl.)—ISBN 0-8157-1851-9 (pa.)
   1. Health care reform—United States.   2. Health care reform—United States—
States.   I. DiIulio, John J.   II. Nathan, Richard R.
RA395.A3M354   1994
362.1 '0973—dc20   94-3690
                                                                              CIP

9 8 7 6 5 4 3 2 1

The paper used in this publication meets the minimum requirements of the American
National Standard for Information Sciences—Permanence of Paper for Printed Library Materials, ANSI Z39.48-1984.

Set in Garamond #3

Composition by Harlowe Typography, Inc., Cottage City, Maryland

Printed by R.R. Donnelley and Sons, Co., Harrisonburg, Virginia

ℬ THE BROOKINGS INSTITUTION

The Brookings Institution is an independent organization devoted to nonpartisan research, education, and publication in economics, government, foreign policy, and the social sciences generally. Its principal purposes are to aid in the development of sound public policies and to promote public understanding of issues of national importance.

The Institution was founded on December 8, 1927, to merge the activities of the Institute for Government Research, founded in 1916, the Institute of Economics, founded in 1922, and the Robert Brookings Graduate School of Economics and Government, founded in 1924.

The Board of Trustees is responsible for the general administration of the Institution, while the immediate direction of the policies, program, and staff is vested in the President, assisted by an advisory committee of the officers and staff. The by-laws of the Institution state: "It is the function of the Trustees to make possible the conduct of scientific research, and publication, under the most favorable conditions, and to safeguard the independence of the research staff in the pursuit of their studies and in the publication of the results of such studies. It is not a part of their function to determine, control, or influence the conduct of particular investigations or the conclusions reached."

The President bears final responsibility for the decision to publish a manuscript as a Brookings book. In reaching his judgment on the competence, accuracy, and objectivity of each study, the President is advised by the director of the appropriate research program and weighs the views of a panel of expert outside readers who report to him in confidence on the quality of the work. Publication of a work signifies that it is deemed a competent treatment worthy of public consideration but does not imply endorsement of conclusions or recommendations.

The Institution maintains its position of neutrality on issues of public policy in order to safeguard the intellectual freedom of the staff. Hence interpretations or conclusions in Brookings publications should be understood to be solely those of the authors and should not be attributed to the Institution, to its trustees, officers, or other staff members, or to the organizations that support its research.

Board of Trustees

James A. Johnson
Chairman

Leonard Abramson
Ronald J. Arnault
Rex J. Bates
A. W. Clausen
John L. Clendenin
D. Ronald Daniel
Walter Y. Elisha
Stephen Friedman

William H. Gray III
Vartan Gregorian
Teresa Heinz
Samuel Hellman
Warren Hellman
Thomas W. Jones
Vernon E. Jordan, Jr.
James A. Joseph
Breene M. Kerr
Thomas G. Labrecque

Donald F. McHenry
Bruce K. MacLaury
David O. Maxwell
Constance Berry Newman
Maconda Brown O'Connor
Samuel Pisar
David Rockefeller, Jr.
Michael P. Schulhof
Robert H. Smith
John D. Zeglis
Ezra K. Zilkha

Honorary Trustees

Elizabeth E. Bailey
Vincent M. Barnett, Jr.
Barton M. Biggs
Louis W. Cabot
Edward W. Carter
Frank T. Cary
William T. Coleman, Jr.
Kenneth W. Dam
Bruce B. Dayton
Douglas Dillon
Charles W. Duncan, Jr.
Robert F. Erburu

Robert D. Haas
Andrew Heiskell
Roger W. Heyns
Roy M. Huffington
Nannerl O. Keohane
James T. Lynn
William McC. Martin, Jr.
Robert S. McNamara
Mary Patterson McPherson
Arjay Miller
Donald S. Perkins

J. Woodward Redmond
Charles W. Robinson
James D. Robinson III
Howard D. Samuel
B. Francis Saul II
Ralph S. Saul
Henry B. Schacht
Robert Brookings Smith
Morris Tanenbaum
John C. Whitehead
James D. Wolfensohn

Foreword

IN THE DEBATE on health care, policymakers and the public have been deluged with information and arguments about competing plans and proposals. But information is not knowledge, and arguments are not necessarily insights.

This publication of the Brookings Center for Public Management neither analyzes nor endorses any particular health care reform proposal. Instead, it offers all those engaged in this historic debate—legislators, journalists, average citizens—a timely reminder about the difficulties of translating federal policy rhetoric into state and local administrative action. Each of the proposed major health care reforms poses significant administrative challenges and opportunities. This volume sounds an alarm for federal policymakers to anticipate these administrative issues by fully coming to grips with the tremendous differences among state health care systems.

This book is based on a project begun in 1993 with support from the Robert Wood Johnson Foundation. A series of seminars and conferences held at the Nelson A. Rockefeller Institute of Government, the public policy research arm of the State University of New York at Albany, resulted in published articles and working papers written in close consultation with health policy officials from a group of states that represent the full range and complexity of state health care systems.

The Rockefeller Institute sponsors the National Commission on the State and Local Public Service, led by William F. Winter, chairman of the Advisory Commission on Intergovernmental Relations and former governor of Mississippi. In 1993 the commission issued its first report on state and local public service reform, as well as a report on health care reform that focused on the role of state governments. Building on its health report, the commission conducted a seminar in Albany last November on the implementation of health care reform as viewed from the states. Officials from seven states—California, Florida, Mississippi, Minnesota, New York, Texas, and Washington—joined a core group of public management and health policy experts for a close look at the Health Security Act proposed by President Bill Clinton. The lead participants, joined by state experts, continued their work in conjunction with the Brookings Center for Public Management. In April 1994, Brookings released a report based on chapter 1 of the present volume.

The editors wish to thank the following participants in the Albany conference: Gary Clarke, vice president, Medicaid Operations, PCA Century and Family Health Plans of Florida; Alton Cobb, former director, Mississippi State Health Department; DeAnn Friedholm, state medicaid director, Texas Health and Human Services Commission; David Maxwell-Jolly, consultant, California Senate Appropriations Committee; Mary Kennedy, senior health policy advisor, Minnesota Department of Health; Michael Hansen, staff director, Committee on Health Care, Florida House of Representatives; Nanette Schroeder, director, Health Care Delivery Systems, Minnesota Department of Health; Margaret Stanley, administrator, Health Care Authority, Washington State; Raymond Sweeney, director, Office of Health Systems Management, New York State Department of Health; Helen Wetherbee, executive director, Division of Medicaid, Mississippi Department of Health; and Paula Wilson, executive deputy commissioner, New York State Department of Health. Sara Sibley Lundine, consultant to the Rockefeller Institute, and Susan O'Loughlin, deputy administrator of policy and program development, Health Care Authority, Washington State, also participated at Brookings. The editors also owe a profound debt to Carey R. Macdonald for her work on the volume and are deeply grateful to Cindy Terrels for assisting with the project. Nancy Davidson and James R. Schneider edited the manuscript, Jeanne C. Moody prepared the index, and Susan R. Woollen prepared the manuscript for typesetting.

The views expressed in this volume are those of the authors and should not be attributed to the persons or organizations whose assistance is acknowledged, or to the trustees, officers, or other staff members of the Brookings Institution.

BRUCE K. MAC LAURY
President

July 1994
Washington, D.C.

Contents

Introduction

John J. DiIulio, Jr., and Richard P. Nathan

OVER THE past few years, two fundamental truths have emerged about health care finance in the United States. First, the system is in bad shape. Some citizens have no health insurance at all, while others with insurance have a difficult time negotiating the system. Second, costs are spiraling and rules are choking the management of health care finance. Reform is needed. But what kind of reform should be enacted? And what policies can make reform work?

Major health care reform plans now being debated in Congress are competing to guarantee health coverage for all Americans and to bring spiraling costs under control. Naturally, supporters of each of the half-dozen or so proposals argue that their plan can best achieve both goals while maintaining or improving the quality of care. But how? The consensus on broad policy goals has given way to a debate over who should pay and how to manage the system. Much of the early critical commentary on President Clinton's health plan, for example, has focused on its administrative complexity.

Our purpose in this book is not to enter the battle over which health care plan to pass. The nation has reached a point at which some health care reform is inevitable. In fact, it is already under way. We argue here that policymakers have an obligation not only to conceive the best policy but also to increase the chances that it will work. As Herbert Kaufman said more than thirty years ago, "Policy is enunciated in rhetoric; it is realized in action."[1] Making it work will require sustained effort, from the earliest stages of policymaking, to identify and solve the critical management problems. We offer a framework for how to do this.

Swift and simultaneous reforms of health insurance coverage, care delivery systems, cost control mechanisms, and medical education will not be easy and may well be impossible. Even the most incremental national plans that promise phased-in reforms but gloss over the political and budgetary realities of policy implementation are bound to get lost in the administrative maze of public, private, and nonprofit organizations that now finance and deliver health care to most Americans.

Of course, policymakers at all levels of government routinely enact new policies or recast old ones without thinking through how the policies can best be put into action or whether, in fact, they can be implemented at all. Lawmakers often establish broad (and not infrequently unreachable) goals and delegate to federal bureaucracies, state and local governments, or, increasingly, private contractors the task of making it all work. Lawmakers have especially tended to devise national policies without fashioning the administrative means to achieve them or anticipating the management problems likely to attend them.

The policy decisions in any health care plan will become real only when they shape action. The administrative success or failure of health care reform, in the end, will define it. Americans have in the past been disappointed by program after program whose results have not measured up to their promises. Health care reform promises to be the biggest single domestic policy innovation in American history. Given its breathtaking scope—health care spending accounts for one-seventh of the American economy—and the utter dependence of many on its success— sick people cannot afford to wait until management problems are cured first—a sound administrative course must be set right from the beginning.

The Role of the States

It would be a mistake to overlook federalism as a critical dimension of national health care reform. Planners must think clearly about the roles of the states—politically, governmentally, legally, and culturally— in the workings of ever more complex governmental systems. Federalism is not a relic of earlier days to be preserved only in unsophisticated introductory government textbooks.

The strength of American federalism is its ability to reconcile unity and diversity in a way that adapts to new social, economic, and technological conditions by means of changes in the roles of different levels of government. As in the current health debate, this adjustment process typically involves the allocation of functions between the national government and the states.

There are three basic aspects of every governmental function: financing it, setting policy for it, and administering it. The redistributive purpose of health care reform justifies a substantial financial role for the national government to spread the burden. With this burden spreading, it is logical that the national government should also determine much of the policy. But the Catch-22 is the third dimension, administration. The national role can be substantial for finance and policymaking, but administrative responsibilities are primarily assigned to the states.

Most plans involve a major role for the national government in determining the hospital and medical benefits to be provided. Most of these plans then turn to the states (some without much specification or clear conceptualization) to set up the administrative machinery to channel benefits to the ultimate customers.

At this stage, policymakers typically make other assignments to the states. States are given the biggest role under most plans to deal with cost containment, as in the Clinton plan, which gives them responsibility for setting the boundaries (a nearly impossible job) and overseeing the activities of regional alliances. Other plans call these entities purchasing cooperatives, and they are of varying degrees of obligation. However, most plans rely on the market-making and regulatory role of state-supervised regional entities to contain costs.

Not only are the states called upon to fulfill these unenviable responsibilities, but they must do so in a way that maintains the quality of care. They are also expected to collect reams of new data, explain them carefully to the public, and take disciplinary action if quality-of-care standards are violated. No doubt some of these duties are seen by the authors of the health care reform plans as things that will somehow be worked out once the financing and the basic policy parameters are set in place.

But there are questions that must be addressed. States are already the administrative agents of federal and state policy under medicaid. They also have major responsibilities for licensing and regulating health professions and financing and administering educational programs for them. And they also regulate insurance and health care providers. A decade ago, Drew Altman and Douglas Morgan emphasized the shared role of governments in health-related matters.[2] Although they depicted the federal government as "the single most important force," they also described in detail what they called "a rediscovery of the importance of the role of state and local governments."

> Broadly speaking, the health-related activities of state and local government are: traditional public health, including health monitoring, sanitation, and disease control; the financing and delivery of personal health services including medicaid, mental health, and direct delivery through public hospitals and health departments; environmental protection, including protection against man-made environmental and occupational hazards; and the regulation of the providers of medical care through certificate-of-need and state rate setting as well as licensing and other functions.[3]

A new health care system should be a federal-state partnership with the federal government as the senior partner. But by no means are state responsibilities trivial. States will need to monitor and control costs; establish and oversee health alliances, if used; foster the development of integrated health plans, certify their eligibility, and ensure their financial solvency; ensure adequate access for all eligible populations and assist with financing health care for the poor; implement insurance reforms; and implement malpractice reforms.[4]

The federalism strategy we advocate is to move first and fastest with the states that are most advanced in a way that takes account of their administrative structures and fits with the programs they have in place, working toward the ultimate goals of the new system. Some states are ready, notably Washington and Minnesota, among the states studied by the National Commission on the State and Local Public Service (the sample included California, Florida, Minnesota, Mississippi, New York, Texas, and Washington). Washington and Minnesota need assistance from the federal government to put reforms in place in a way that fits with the new national design. Other states are unlikely to be able to move as quickly. Mississippi and Texas, among the seven states in the sample, have the longest way to go. They will need to be provided incentives and requirements on a schedule that takes account of the barriers they face.

Recognizing states that are ahead of the others as needing to be helped rather than pushed has deep roots in federalism theory. Over time in American federalism, there has been a cyclicality in the relative roles of the national government and state governments, with the swing variable in this cyclical pattern being political ideology. In conservative periods the role of state governments has been strengthened; in liberal or pro-government periods, the responsibilities of the national government have grown. In liberal periods those who favor increased government activity often find that it is efficient to lobby for their interests at one place, the center. In conservative periods the proponents of increased governmental activity have fewer opportunities; they have to try to get changes adopted wherever they can. Pro-government lobbying activities are thus focused on those states in which there is support for a new or stronger role for the public sector. As is the case today in health care, states—not all states, but many—have been centers of activism and innovation in domestic affairs.[5]

At the national level the institutional design for a new health care system should consist of two main parts: adopting a basic policy framework for the new system, and setting up a process to adjust this policy framework as it is implemented. The implementation process should be adaptive, building on lessons from experience as it is gained. This is especially important for cost containment.

The Clinton plan establishes a national health board. Other plans have similar central management structures. But how will this machinery work? A national board with the states represented directly or in an advisory capacity could have the power to modify the new system by sending regular (perhaps annual) revised plans to Congress. Authority also could be included for interstate compacts so that some states (particularly less populous ones) could form a consortium to implement the new system and regional purchasing cooperatives could be created across state lines in large metropolitan areas.

In reviews of the revised plans, this adjustment mechanism could work like the military base-closing commission. Congress could be required to consider revisions proposed by a national health board as a package; they could send the plan back to the board, but not change it. There have been three base-closing commissions that worked this way since Congress enacted the Base Closure and Realignment Act of 1988. Although this has not been a politically simon-pure process, it has been a way to bring expertise to bear on a difficult set of issues and provide a needed measure of political insulation for politicians who know what they want to do, but see the task as a "third-rail" issue (one that is too hot to touch) for the officeholders directly affected by the adjustment process.

One can think of this base-closing approach as a designated driver system for government. We know where we want to go, but we have some bad habits. You take us there, but drive carefully. Setting up and implementing a new national health care system that includes strong provisions for cost containment requires such a mechanism for driving carefully. Political leaders must make the hard choices and set the country on course to the destination, but we will need all the ingenuity and skill we can bring to the process of getting there.

To summarize, new national legislation should be viewed in a way that gives attention to three principles of federalism about how a new system will affect the states:

—The new law should reflect what states can really do: when, how, and in what sequence.

—It should reflect clear thinking about how feedback from the states will be factored into the implementation process. (The new health care system is bound to be revised frequently, probably every year.)

—It should assure that policy changes do not disrupt ongoing reforms in the states that are already most advanced in reforming their health care systems.

Woodrow Wilson said in 1908 that "the question of the relation of the states to the federal government is the cardinal question of our constitutional system." It cannot be settled, said Wilson, by "one generation, because it is a question of growth, and every successive stage of our political and economic development gives it a new aspect, makes it a new question."[6] Wilson's "cardinal question" as it applies to health policy is sure to be prominent for a long time, not just as new laws are enacted but throughout the process of setting up the machinery to implement them.

Summary of the Book

Together with Donald F. Kettl, in chapter 1 we summarize the main ideas of the present volume. Our message is that before federal policy-makers reinvent the nation's health care system they need to rediscover the states. Drawing on the health policy and administrative experiences of seven states, we discuss competing approaches to health care reform and offer six working principles that, if followed, would help produce an administratively sound national health care reform plan. The most basic precondition for administrative success is to define and delineate clearly the federal and state roles. We outline how this may be done.

In chapter 2, James R. Tallon, Jr., and Lawrence D. Brown discuss the functions and forms of health care alliances and the aspects of federalism they involve. Moving beyond the dead-end debate over the administrative complexity of competing plans, they demonstrate that, short of a single-payer system or another approach in which government insures the entire citizenry, new administrative forms will be needed to execute six functions: concert purchaser leverage, avert the selection of only people who are preferred risks, empower and inform consumers, administer and disburse subsidies, collect and allocate premiums, and negotiate and persuade. These functions, they reason, are indispensable to a successful refashioning of health insurance markets that are clearly in disarray. The regional health alliances proposed by the Clinton administration may or may not be the answer, but some such mechanisms are essential to various species of health care reform policy.

The primary dilemma for federal and state policymakers, Tallon and Brown comment, "is whether alliances will be able to perform these functions. Who will run them day to day, and how do states prepare for the challenges of staffing?" Their view from the states on alliances is sobering but hopeful: "A federally mandated choice between health alliances and a single-payer model makes little sense when neither option fits well in two-thirds or more of the states," and "the sooner policymakers dispel illusions of automaticity in implementation, the better. The structural issues surrounding alliances are complex and intensely political. . . . Establishing and monitoring alliances and their relation with health plans demands significantly upgraded state managerial capacities: more and better-trained staff in health and insurance departments; more and better data and the management information systems to process them; and more sophisticated and sustained dialogues among state health officials, alliance boards and staffs, and managers of health plans."

Echoing the broader themes of the rest of the volume, Tallon and Brown make the case that health alliances can work, but only if the necessary administrative forethought goes into their design and execution. Likewise, in chapter 3, James W. Fossett analyzes the issue of cost containment and rate setting. As he shows, except for the few states that have been engaged in all-payer hospital rate regulation on a more or less regular basis since the late 1970s, state experience with cost containment has been limited and uneven. This limited experience and the considerable controversy over expanding it "suggest that the successful institutionalization of cost containment will be among the most difficult political and administrative tasks for any national plan."

Fossett examines two generic cost containment methods—expenditure regulation, practiced in many European countries, and revenue regulation, contemplated in the Clinton proposal and recently begun in Minnesota and Washington State. Many difficult administrative challenges await any significant effort at cost containment. To cite just one, the states' ability to measure or monitor expenditures currently ranges from limited to nonexistent. A few states maintain hospital discharge databases, but these systems vary greatly in quality.

Fossett's analysis underlines the potential legal and political barriers to effective cost containment. Politically and administratively successful cost containment is likely to require a long start-up period in which the basic organizational framework of reform is put into place and efforts at developing appropriate data and measurement systems are initiated. This beginning would be followed by a slow and uneven but increasingly steady pattern of incremental reduction in the rate of cost growth. But this pattern conflicts with the budget process, which requires that additional expenditures must be financed with more certainty over a much shorter time.

Devising and administering effective cost containment policies is one huge challenge of reform. But as Frank J. Thompson demonstrates in chapter 4, implementing quality assurance policies in a universal health care system may be an even bigger challenge. Using the quality assurance provisions of the Clinton plan to illustrate his argument, Thompson analyzes three sets of dilemmas: fashioning meaningful and consumer-friendly "report cards" on health plans and providers; promulgating medical practice guidelines based on research on scientific outcomes; and creating channels for consumers to voice their views and grievances about the health insurance and health care delivery systems that affect them.

Few states have developed anything like the information technologies and data-based management systems that would be necessary but insufficient administrative conditions for the quality assurance provisions of the Clinton plan to work. More broadly, on a large number of health care problems and matters of medical practice, there is no scientific consensus. Thus, Thompson notes, a swarm of political and legal problems awaits those who would attempt to implement report cards and other quality assurance measures.

The Clinton plan, for example, via its proposed national quality management council mandates the development and use of several dozen performance indicators within a few years of the plan's adoption. But officials in the New York State Department of Health wanted to develop a handful of indicators for health maintenance organizations (HMOs) focused on preventive care (prenatal visits, immunizations, mammographies). After five months of negotiations with the HMOs, they had reached agreement on just one indicator for one type of preventive measure (immunizations). As a top state health official quoted by Thompson observes, "At that rate, we will get to 50 indicators [by] the time none of us are around to appreciate it." Mustering scientific claims for the validity of report cards, Thompson adds, "would not be easy for defenders, given the gross limits to knowledge concerning how to develop valid summary measures of the quality of medical care. The report card could come to reflect the political muscle of various groups of disease advocates as much as it did more scientific assessments of quality."

Still, Thompson does not give report cards and other quality assurance efforts a failing grade. Rather, he concludes by suggesting how to make them work by deferring to the states, setting realistic measurement targets, and proceeding incrementally. In some instances, "a decentralized, deregulated, phased-in approach to quality assurance," he writes, "would allow the federal government to learn from various state experiences. . . . In sum, proponents of quality assurance under comprehensive health care reform cannot escape the challenge of implementing programs through the federal system. This challenge would be significant but, sensibly approached, far from insurmountable."

Regardless of what type of health plan they favor, most reformers agree that the nation has too many medical specialists, too few general practitioners, and too many medically underserved communities. Today, less than one-third of all physicians are generalists, and less than 20 percent of first-year residents choose generalist practice. The distribution of America's medical work force has been blamed for everything from rising costs driven by high-technology specialized medicine to problems of access caused by the failure of doctors to locate in poor and rural areas of the country. Moreover, a change in the composition and practice patterns of America's medical work force is presupposed by managed care plans in which primary care doctors are to serve as the administrative linchpins, providing clients with needed basic care while guiding them away from unnecessary specialty treatment.

In chapter 5, Michael S. Sparer examines the administrative dynamics of altering the nation's medical work force. The Clinton plan, for example, would require that by 1998 at least 55 percent of all entering medical residents be generalists. To even begin to achieve that goal,

Sparer shows, would require a virtual revolution in the way that medical schools and teaching hospitals operate. And previous federal and state efforts to alter the medical work force give very little cause for optimism. Indeed, Sparer estimates that even if the institutional change were easy to accomplish, the medical training pipeline is so long that producing a ratio of 50 percent generalists and 50 percent specialists would still take almost fifty years.

But there are silver linings. For example, Sparer reports that although the percentage of generalist physicians has declined precipitously between 1960 and today, the actual ratio of generalists-to-population has remained relatively constant (at approximately 75 generalists per 100,000 population). There is, he suggests, tremendous interstate variation in medical work force problems, with some states relatively well off in terms of both the ratio of generalists to specialists and the geographic distribution of doctors, and other states (most notably in his analysis Texas) with large numbers of medically underserved citizens. On balance, the more pressing nationwide medical work force maldistribution problem, he finds, is the geographic one. This problem, he concludes, can be addressed by strong federal action, much of it through established administrative channels, including the National Health Service Corps.

In chapter 6, John J. DiIulio, Jr., Donald F. Kettl, and Gerald Garvey place the implementation, management, and federalism challenges of health care reform in the context of other national policy initiatives (welfare, environmental protection, youth and families, crime, and transportation). The literature on policy implementation, they suggest, is a litany of missed opportunities and spoiled hopes. But health care reform need not become yet another chapter in this history of administrative failures. "Perhaps the single most instructive administrative analogy," they suggest, "is to the quarter-century-old attempt to reform the nation's environmental protection system." In the course of drawing this analogy, they cite one study that found major and generally undesirable differences in how EPA-funded state pollution prevention programs actually work. Their main contention is that the nation's environmental reform effort would be much stronger today had the architects of federal pollution prevention and other policies taken pains from the beginning to wire administrative success into their plans by developing the necessary administrative guidance and oversight capacity within the federal service, taking stock of the varying administrative capacities of the states, and linking management responsibilities with budgetary muscle. It is not too late, they conclude, to do these things in the area of health care reform.

As Martha Derthick concluded in one of her landmark studies, "policymaking neglects administration," and "the most cherished structural features of American government pose obstacles to good administration." One such feature is federalism, which "fragments administrative structures, necessitating the construction of elaborate arrangements for intergovernmental cooperation."[7] In the concluding chapter of the present volume, Lawrence D. Brown suggests that, viewed from the states, health care reform is doable, but only if national policymakers do not attempt to do all good things at once, and only if they anticipate the administrative opportunities and obstacles posed by federalism. Five areas, he argues, "are especially important to workable state implementation of national health reform": regulation, information, planning, negotiation, and reorganization. "Implementing programmatic details and managing institutional complexity," he notes, "are well down the list of priorities of most of those promoting health reform." As he concludes, "The politics of federal policymaking often defeat orderly federalism and regularly confer in the states the worst of both worlds— tight federal constraints that inhibit innovation and responsiveness plus broad delegations of authority that expect states to solve problems that send federal leaders running for cover."

This should be obvious. Translating national health care reform policy rhetoric into effective state-level administrative action is bound to require lots of human energy, financial investment, legal maneuvering, untold acts of bureaucratic cooperation, and untold measures of political forbearance. But the post–World War II history of federal policymaking, including the contemporary debates and proposals over health care reform, tells us that, when it comes to issues of policy implementation, management, and federalism, action the least bit respectful of this obvious administrative reality would be exceptional, a rare mark of administrative maturity in a system in which policy implementation is too often a political afterthought and public management too often a political orphan.

1 ||| Administrative Principles

John J. DiIulio, Jr., Richard P. Nathan,
and Donald F. Kettl

SIX WORKING PRINCIPLES must underpin the effort to create
an administratively sound national health care reform policy. First, any
health care reform plan will be complex. What matters is not how
complex the system is, but how well it works. Complexity and work-
ability are not necessarily related. Second, reforms have often sacrificed
administrative simplicity to realize other values. The effort to protect
program responsiveness, ease of access, and other desirable attributes
will likely lead to health care reform through administrative hybrids—
federal-state, public-private. Third, in these hybrid organizations the
states will be crucial participants. Understanding their functions and
differing capacities is critical to successful management. Fourth, because
different states have different capacities, different plans impose very
different administrative tasks. Success will require matching administrative methods to the tasks. Fifth, the federal and state governments
will have very different functions in health care reform. Reform will
require delimiting a coherent division of labor as those responsibilities
are defined and the capacity to fulfill them is built. Finally, the steps
required to reform health care cannot be accomplished at once. Planners
will have to determine what needs to be done first, what can be left
until later, and what should not be attempted at all.

No Escape from Administrative Complexity

Critics of the Clinton health plan have charged that because it is too
complex, it should not be passed. This charge, however, focuses on the

wrong objective. Complexity is not the standard by which any health plan ought to be judged. Far more important is whether it is likely to achieve the desired results.

Every day, Americans deal with systems of remarkable complexity without giving them a second thought. The steps involved in transactions at an automatic teller machine would generate a complex diagram. The nation's air traffic control system requires imposing interconnections of people, organizations, and technology. The complexity of these systems does not matter; results do. What matters to people is that when they encounter the system, it produces results without imposing unacceptable transaction costs.

The current U.S. health care system fails this test. It does not cover all Americans and it creates managerial migraines for everyone who encounters it. Billions of dollars are lost because of waste, fraud, and abuse in the processing of medicare claims. There is also an unacceptable human and financial toll even when the system is working as it was meant to. Everyone—sick people and their families, physicians and their staffs, employers who contribute to their workers' health insurance, hospital executives and government overseers—must confront maddening and expensive paperwork, regulatory restrictions, and inflexibility.[1]

For instance, the federal government funds care for the old, the disabled, and the poor through medicare and medicaid. Nearly all the care, however, comes through for-profit and nonprofit physicians and hospitals. Intermediaries manage most of the money. More than eighty private contractors handle the claims for medicare, and the states are responsible for arranging for and administering about half of medicaid expenses. The federal government, in addition, runs one of the nation's largest hospital systems through the Department of Veterans Affairs. The VA has had serious problems in managing its system effectively. Employer-provided health care insurance for employees also runs into snarls of bureaucracy. Efforts by employers and insurers alike have produced a complex of review organizations, health purchasing cooperatives, prepaid health plans, and other hybrid organizations. The regulatory responsibilities of state governments have escalated as they have launched their own programs to ensure the integrity of private insurance plans, help solve the problem of the uninsured, and control their own spiraling medicaid costs. Finally some citizens purchase their own insurance and have to cope with the complexity on their own.

The administrative failure of the status quo is one of the most important reasons for reform. The system's ungovernability is expensive for everyone. It encourages restrictions on coverage and the transferability of insurance. It interferes with physicians as they try to practice medicine and with patients who need care. In sum, the administrative status quo is riddled with management problems that drive costs up and quality down.

The illustrations are many. Fraud, waste, and abuse plague the medicare program. According to the General Accounting Office, billions of dollars leak out of the program because of management difficulties. The Department of Veterans Affairs loses millions of dollars each year because of its inability to verify that veterans meet income limitations for service. State governments have had their own problems in managing medicaid. Federal rules limit their discretion in assigning care. Nursing home costs in particular drive spending inexorably upward. State managers have struggled to be innovative in a program whose federal mandates leave them little maneuvering room.[2] In the private sector the administrative costs of individual and small-group plans can account for up to 40 percent of the costs of claims. In short, as studies of health care in many nations consistently point out, Americans spend far more to run their health care system than citizens of other nations.

It is, frankly, hard to imagine any reform that attempts to alter the structure of one-seventh of the American economy that would not be complex. But in assessing the complexity of reform proposals, there are three critical questions. Is the plan more or less complex than the status quo? Is it worth creating more complexity—new organizations or government rules, for instance—in exchange for greater social benefits such as guaranteed universal access of all citizens to health care? Finally, can complex health care reforms be engineered to be more user friendly?

These questions need to be answered now so that it will not be necessary to hold hearings or write studies a decade from now about why some aspect of the plan has failed. An analogy may help to illustrate this crucial point. In 1970 America launched a major national effort to clean up its environment. Administratively, the effort involved the states and a broad array of private contractors. Twenty-four years later, few are satisfied with what has been achieved, and we are still working the bugs out of that system. National health care reform is an even bigger administrative task than environmental cleanup. And the United States is seeking to do far more in far less time. To demand quick results without first drawing an administrative chart is to cruise directly into the path of hundreds of managerial icebergs.

The lesson: the ability to produce results, far more than the ability to craft a simple, politically acceptable plan, will ultimately determine the quality of health care in the United States. This, in turn, will shape the public's confidence in the government's ability not merely to promise but to deliver.

Reliance on Hybrid Organizations

Because administrative simplicity of proposed plans has been a touchstone for judging health care reform, reformers and their critics have looked at each plan's organization to assess the odds that it will work. Some reformers have argued that a single-payer system is best because it establishes a simple connection between government and health care recipients. Others have contended that any government involvement will inevitably create needless complexity and an endlessly expanding bureaucracy. Indeed, some of the harshest attacks on the Clinton administration's plans have come from critics charging that the proposed mixed public-private system could never work.

The easiest way to achieve administrative simplicity is to follow the old precept of unity of command: assign administrative responsibilities to a single entity and set up a straightforward chain of command. That, however, is the one approach that any conceivable health reform will not pursue. Indeed, since the creation of the social security program, a national program run by a national agency, every major domestic policy innovation has relied on a hybrid of public and private sector organizations. Medicare claims, for example, are processed through a network of private contractors. The states perform most of the administrative work for the medicaid program. There is no reason to think that a new health care program will be any different.

Any health care program will require substantial administrative machinery to make it work. Eligibility will have to be reviewed, claim forms checked, expenses reimbursed, quality measured. There is no political support for a big government bureaucracy to solve the problem, but neither are government decisionmakers comfortable with allowing private organizations to manage a public program without considerable supervision by public officials. For a generation the federal government has sought to solve complex public problems by working through a dilemma: how to achieve public control without significantly increasing public bureaucracy. The management of any health care reform program will likely rely, as previous public programs have, on a complex partnership between the federal and state governments, and among government and private for-profit and nonprofit organizations.

The lesson: administrative simplicity is not the only value to pursue in health care reform. Responsiveness, competition, oversight by public authority, and the flexibility of private markets will also be important. The management of health care reform is therefore likely to rely on a hybrid system, and the states are likely to be the focus.

State Roles in Health Care Provision

The states have long been important to hybrid systems, and they will be key participants in health care reform. States improve the responsiveness of national programs to local conditions and share the financial and administrative burdens of national programs. Indeed, the more a program's implementation has relied on delegated power to decide details, the more it has relied on the states.

Since the end of World War II, virtually every major domestic policy innovation—from transportation improvements to environmental cleanup, welfare to low-income housing—has involved state and local governments. Federal programs have succeeded only to the degree that these partnerships have been nourished and energized.[3] So it will be with any likely national health care reform. In its review of the governance issues raised by the Clinton plan, the Congressional Budget Office observed that the administration's proposal "would place new responsibilities on the federal and state governments, create a variety of new institutions, and specify a complex flow of resources among those institutions."[4] If federal policymakers are to be effective in reinventing the nation's health care system, they must first rediscover the vital and varied administrative functions of the states in deciding who gets covered and treated, for what, how, by whom, and under what conditions.

The administrative capacities of the states, however, vary widely. When it comes to health care administration, America has a hodgepodge of systems and programs operating under diverse and shifting political, legal, budgetary, and technical constraints. A 1993 report by the General Accounting Office, for example, found wide differences in state regulation of the insurance industry. Before West Virginia Blue Cross failed in 1990, state insurance regulators knew of impending problems but "took little action against the plan because of a lack of resources and regulatory authority." Hawaii, Nevada, and Wyoming spent less than 10 percent of their insurance department budgets on health care regulation; seventeen states spent more than 25 percent. Fourteen states had no actuary on staff or under contract to work on health insurance. Nine did not investigate consumer complaints against insurers. And only a few states reviewed first-time premium rates before they took effect.[5] Administratively, the nation's health care system is a nonsystem. There is little possibility that this can be changed greatly, if at all, by federal fiat, and no possibility whatsoever that it can be changed anytime soon.

Every state is wrestling, with varying speed and success, to initiate reforms to meet state needs. The National Commission on the State and Local Public Service, which studied seven states in Albany in November 1993, found a wide range of experiences in implementing health care reform. Minnesota and Washington are engaged in significant restructurings of their health care systems. California, Florida, and New York are in midcourse, with new laws on the books that promise to lead to meaningful reform. Mississippi and Texas have only just begun to move tentatively and incrementally toward reform.

Because states' experiences and capacities differ so greatly, no one-size-fits-all approach is possible. There is positively no way that Texas, Mississippi, and other states with limited experience could begin to meet the timetables, requirements for insurer alliance structures, certification procedures, quality control mandates, and cost containment responsibilities specified in titles I, II, V, and VIII of the Health Security Act (the Clinton plan). To create the mere rudiments of the regulatory structures called for in most of the plans could take these states years. To implement a program fully would take a decade or longer.

Other states would seem tailor-made for some health reform plans. There would appear to be none more ready for the Clinton plan than Washington State, for instance. But administrative appearances can be very deceiving. Not even Washington, one of the most innovative and experienced states, is a computer into which a disk of the Clinton plan or any plan even remotely like it could be inserted and the programs copied without hitch. Washington's health care reform law, for instance, incorporates group purchasing policies and arrangements, and the state has gained a lot of valuable experience in operating its version of this administrative form. But the employer alliances and purchaser cooperatives called for in the Clinton plan would require more and different responsibilities and operate in different ways from those created in Olympia. The Washington State management information systems would also have to be radically altered to implement the provisions of the Clinton plan.

There are many such mismatches in policy emphasis between the two Washingtons that translate directly into significant differences between the administrative structures contemplated in the national plan and those currently at work in the state (table 1-1). These differences bring up an underappreciated administrative truth. To meet any plan's most basic policy provisions, "undeveloped" states such as Mississippi and Texas would have to build from scratch. Even Washington, Minnesota, and other more "advanced" states would have to rebuild much of their systems. In all cases, adapting to any national plan would demand a great deal of planning time, personnel energy, and expense—more time, energy, and expense than any of the leading national reform plans acknowledges or allows.

Adapting current state systems to new national demands is a major administrative problem that any health care system will have to solve. Because the states are starting from different places with different capacities, uniform results will not be possible anytime soon.

The lesson: the states are likely to be important administrative partners in any health care reform plan. But their capacities to fulfill their responsibilities would vary widely. To achieve success, any reform plan must develop a strategy for moving toward a system that meets national, and uniform, health care goals but that builds on the considerable administrative differences among the states.

Differences in Management Burdens

Like other government programs, health care reform draws on various management tactics and strategies that, when combined, produce the administrative system on which success depends. In health policy the principal management tools are

—direct service delivery, in which the government itself produces a service;

—regulation, in which government rules govern how someone else provides a service;

—information gathering, in which the government collects data on the system;

—institution building, in which the government creates new public or quasi-public organizations to make the system function;

—tax incentives, in which the government uses the tax code to create the incentive for someone to provide a service; and

—subsidies, in which the government pays for a service, or requires others to pay for or subsidize a service, without necessarily providing it.

These methods are sometimes used by the federal government, sometimes by state governments, sometimes in intergovernmental partnerships, and sometimes in complex partnerships with for-profit and nonprofit organizations.

In health care reform it must be remembered that every plan imposes major administrative burdens. No plan could truly be considered administratively simple because the system being reformed is itself both huge and complex. In addition, the administrative requirements vary enormously from plan to plan. Different plans create very different demands on federal and state governments in particular. Rarely do policymakers think carefully about the choices among the policy tools that their proposals imply. But how well the methods are managed will define how well any policy plan will work.

The imposition of major administrative burdens by all six early national proposals (table 1-2) as well as the plans developed later, such as the one put forward by Representative Pete Stark of California, means that they share common concerns.

Consider the management implications of each tool.

Regulation

All health programs will have rules: who pays, who is eligible for benefits, which benefits are covered. They define the characteristics of the system and safeguard its recipients. They minimize waste, fraud, and abuse. They define the responsibilities of providers and give them assurance about how the system will work. Regulation is unavoidable. The key is to make certain that it becomes neither abusive nor excessively costly.

Information Gathering

Less obvious but just as important is the need for information gathering. All plans will require improved information gathering. We cannot know how good a health system is if we cannot look carefully at

Table 1-1. Clinton Plan and the Washington State Health System

Feature	Clinton administration	Washington State

Financing coverage

Feature	Clinton administration	Washington State
Employers	All firms must pay 80% or more of average premium for employees and dependents up to total payroll caps (adjusted for two-income families). Firms with more than 75 workers or average wages greater than $24,000 will pay 7.9% of payroll. Sliding caps for firms with average wages less than $24,000 to a minimum 3.5% if average wages are less than $12,000. Prorated contribution for part-time workers (less than 30 hrs/wk). Mandate phased in through 1998.	All firms must pay at least 50% and not more than 100% of the lowest priced plan premium for employees and dependents. Prorated contribution for part-time workers (less than 30 hrs/wk). Mandate is phased in through 1999, starting with employers with 500 workers or more in 1995.
Individuals and families	Workers pay up to 20% of average premium, more if they choose a costlier plan. Federal subsidies for families or individuals with incomes less than 150% of poverty. Persons who are self-employed or part-year employees will calculate contributions and subsidies according to a separate formula.	All state residents must purchase coverage by 1999. Worker pays difference between employer share (50-100% of lowest priced plan) and actual premium.
Subsidized programs	Federal government subsidizes employer shares above payroll caps. People 65 years or older: medicare or coverage through regional health alliances. Retirees 55-64 years: federal government pays 80% of premiums through alliances. AFDC/SSI beneficiaries: medicaid pays premiums to alliances. Other medicaid beneficiaries: join alliances as individuals.	In 1997, $150 million subsidy pool available to companies with fewer than 25 workers. Business and occupation tax credit proposed by 1997 for 40% or less of dependent coverage costs for firms with fewer than 500 employees. Medicaid funding available for children below 200% of federal poverty. Basic health plan expanded statewide (subsidized premiums) for families below 200% of federal poverty.

Table 1-1   *(continued)*

Feature	Clinton administration	Washington State
Benefits package		
Standard package	Inpatient, outpatient, prescriptions, maternity, prevention, reproductive, hospice, home health, mental health, substance abuse, child dental, home/community based long-term care phased in by 2000; occupational/speech therapy, eye care. Benefits depend on covered services and cost-sharing rules. National board will make implementation decisions at the margins.	By 1995 inpatient, outpatient, prescriptions, prevention, reproductive, short-term skilled nursing, hospice, substance abuse, mental health, child preventive dental. Long-term care integrated by 1999.
Supplemental package	National board defines two supplemental packages that health plans may offer consistent with rules set by the board.	Health plans may offer supplemental packages subject to premium and other regulations.
Group purchasing		
Alliances and cooperatives	By 1997 states must create one or more noncompeting regional alliances as nonprofits or state agencies. Firms with 5,000 or more workers may create corporate alliances; they may operate their own health plans, but must offer at least three plans (at least one plan must be fee-for-service, at least two must not be). All citizens must obtain coverage through an alliance, except those covered by medicare. Alliance functions include enrollment, subsidy management, premium collection/distribution, consumer information, health plan marketing regulation, premium risk management. Alliances may not bear risk.	State commission must designate four noncompeting, nonprofit regional insurance purchasing cooperatives serving 150,000 people or more. Coverage through cooperatives is voluntary for employers and individuals. Cooperatives must offer every health plan in their region. Functions include enrollment, premium collection/distribution, and consumer information. Cooperatives may neither bear risk nor negotiate premiums.

Table 1-1 *(continued)*

Feature	Clinton administration	Washington State
Health plans	Health plans must meet federal standards and be state certified. Plans must offer community-rated premiums (actual premiums will vary according to risk-adjustment criteria defined by board), have annual open enrollment periods, and enroll anyone, regardless of health status or other characteristics. Most alliances must offer at least one fee-for-service/free-choice-of-provider plan, subject to regulation.	Health plans must be state certified and comply with uniform administrative, open enrollment, and maximum community-rated premium rules. Plans must enroll anyone, regardless of health status or other characteristics. Limited dental health plans allowed. Firms with more than 7,000 workers may operate their own health plans subject to same regulation. All employers must offer at least three plans or join a cooperative health plan.
Governance		
Federal government	Seven-member national health board appointed by president refines benefits package, issues rules for and enforces national budget through allocations to regional alliances, approves state plans, creates rules for risk adjustment and proportional premiums for families (versus individuals or couples), creates quality program, and creates advisory committees. Secretaries of Labor and HHS retain substantial regulatory and oversight power. Federal government has default responsibility to set up and run alliances if states do not and to penalize states.	Reform law requires congressional action to allow employer mandate by amending ERISA, and other federal action to allow integration of medicare, medicaid, and (potentially) other federal programs such as CHAMPUS, military health, and federal employees.
State government	States submit implementation plans to national health board, including subsidies administration, health plan certification and regulation, data collection and quality assurance, and establishment and governance of health alliances.	Health Services Commission—insurance commissioner (nonvoting) and five members appointed by governor—defines uniform benefit package and maximum premium, sets health plan certification rules, and creates service effectiveness and other advisory committees.

Table 1-1 *(continued)*

Feature	Clinton administration	Washington State
Cost control	National health board determines a premium target for each alliance. Premium growth will be limited to CPI by 1997. Price competition among plans expected to moderate premium increases. If an alliance's average premium exceeds the target, the board may take action to lower it. Medicare and medicaid spending cuts total $238 billion during 1996-2000. Low and high out-of-pocket cost benefits packages will be offered. Administrative savings are attained through uniform claims, data reporting, and payment standards. Billing above schedule is banned for both alliance providers and medicare.	State commision, with legislative consent, sets maximum premium for uniform benefits package in 1995. Price competition among plans is expected to moderate premium increases. The law requires that growth rate of the maximum premium be reduced 2 percentage points each year from historical growth levels until rate is no more than that of per capita state personal income. Uniform benefits package includes copayments and deductibles, except for preventive services. Administrative savings attained through uniform claims, data reporting, and billing standards set by state commission.
Public health	Plan includes additional financial support for core state and local public health functions, strategies to address high-priority public health problems, and federal public health capacity.	Reform law requires a public health improvement plan to enhance state and local core and high-priority public health functions. State commission must coordinate policymaking with public health agencies.
Other	Contingency legal fees are to be capped at 33.5%. Requirements for use of alternative dispute resolution. Health plans will be required to contract with academic medical centers for certain disease treatments. Federal government will set new antitrust rules. Provisions for integrating existing federal programs with the new structure.	Reform law requires studies to integrate workers' compensation, long-term care, CHAMPUS, veterans, and federal employees. Insurance commissioner must implement short-term insurance reforms. Mandatory mediation of malpractice claims.

Source: University of Washington Health Policy Analysis Program, *Washington Health*, 1993.

Table 1-2.   Health Care Reform Management Techniques Used in Six Reform Plans, by Implementing Level of Government

Plan	Direct government administration	Regulation	Tax incentives	Institution building	Information gathering
Clinton administration					
Federal	No	Yes	No	Yes	Yes
State	No	Yes	No	Yes	Yes
McDermott-Wellstone					
Federal	No	Yes	No	Yes	Yes
State	No	Yes	No	No	No
Michael-Lott					
Federal	No	Yes	No	No	Yes
State	No	Yes	No	No	Yes
Cooper-Breaux					
Federal	No	Yes	No	Yes	Yes
State	No	Yes	No	Yes	Yes
Stearns-Nickles					
Federal	No	Yes	Yes	No	Yes
State	No	Yes	No	No	Yes
Thomas-Chafee					
Federal	No	Yes	Yes	No	Yes
State	No	Yes	No	Yes	Yes

Source: Derived from Melvina Ford and others, *Summary Comparison of Major Health Care Reform Bills* (Congressional Research Service, 1994).

how it works. At the same time, any system involving all citizens and so much money will threaten with a tidal wave of paper anyone who wants to examine its performance. If the paper is not kept in check and the right information remains ungathered, governance of the system will be handicapped and the program will become susceptible to abuse. Medicare, for example, has mistakenly paid billions of dollars in claims actually covered by other insurance plans. The program's managers could not sort out the data to avoid the problem. Private insurers fight a similar battle, although their struggles are not as open to public view. Physicians, however, complain about the paperwork burden of insurance programs, and few hospital patients can make sense of their bills. Information gathering and processing is the Achilles' heel of health care reform. The General Accounting Office has found that "agency after agency still lacks critical information needed to analyze programmatic issues, manage agency resources, control expenditures, and demonstrate measurable results. Moreover, the government is falling farther behind the private sector in using information technology to streamline its operations and improve service to the public."[6]

Modernizing the health care system will require modernizing government's information systems. Without this step, no health care reform can succeed.

Institution Building

Many of the plans require hybrid governmental or quasi-governmental organizations to link public funders and private providers. Whether these organizations are called alliances, purchasing cooperatives, or something else, they are new entities with new functions. Some might be government agencies and carry government's full force. Others might be nonprofit and act as agents of the government at a boundary between it and the private sector. Still others might be profit-making organizations.

Whatever the choice of structure, if the plan requires structures, they will have to be built, in some cases from scratch. The *New York Times* metaphorically calls them giant shopping malls in which shoppers can make individual health care choices.[7] But new malls need access roads, and the stores have to be constructed, their shelves stocked, and cash registers installed. In some states without much experience, preparing the land just to start construction will require a major effort.

The organizations need to have enough of a bureaucracy to get the job done without creating one that gets in the way, reducing efficiency and driving up costs. Citizens need to be sure the hybrids are responsive to their needs. Health care providers will want to make sure their interests are considered. And because government, both federal and state, will pay a large share of the costs of any system, each level will have a strong interest in ensuring that the public's money is well spent. These concerns are in part administrative, to ensure effectiveness; in part financial, to ensure efficiency; and in part political, to ensure control and responsiveness.

Designing these structures will require a skilled administrative hand. It will also require imaginative approaches to enduring problems of public law. Where will government's authority rest? Who bears legal liability for decisions? The more complicated the administrative hybrid, the more work will be required to construct a new system of administrative law that clearly sets legal responsibility for decisions under health care reform. The litigation that has surrounded environmental policy suggests just how difficult and contentious this can be.

Other proposals require government to significantly expand existing organizations. In the states that have already experimented with health care reform, experience has varied considerably. Even the most successful efforts depend on new kinds of organizations—and these organizations are working at the limits of their design. To expand their responsibilities will challenge management severely. To create such organizations where they have not previously existed will inevitably prove difficult for hard-pressed states. One way or another, health care reform will require innovative thinking in institutional design.

Tax Incentives

Plans requiring the creation of new organizations rely less heavily on tax incentives; those building on tax incentives depend less heavily on creating new organizations. Even health care proposals that rely more heavily on influencing decisions through changes in the tax code will require skilled administration. The Internal Revenue Service will have to make its rules clear. Individuals and corporations will have to be able to wade through the rules to file their returns, and the agency will then have to be able to monitor the returns to ensure that taxpayers make only legitimate use of the code. But the IRS is struggling with an unreliable information system that hinders its ability to monitor tax returns. Pursuing health care reform even through minimal intervention in the economy will put big burdens on the agency. Indeed, some plans would require major innovations in how it operates. But as the GAO concluded, during the past quarter-century the agency "has twice tried and failed to modernize its antiquated tax-processing system. Unreliable and unresponsive, this system impedes the IRS' ability to collect and account for about a trillion dollars in revenue."[8]

Subsidies

A special problem for all the health care plans is how to cover low-income people who cannot pay for health care on their own. All plans rely on both federal and state subsidies. At a minimum, they anticipate that citizens receiving government-financed medicare and medicaid will continue to receive government health benefits. Some of the plans also provide federal subsidies for health insurance for the poor, small companies, or the uninsured. Creating and managing these subsidies will require substantial administrative work. Most plans envision some federal subsidy to ensure that the poor will not be overlooked. To manage such a subsidy, however, requires that difficult questions be answered first. Who will qualify for subsidies? What standards will be used to make this determination? Who will interpret the standards and make the decisions? And, in the end, who will pay for the coverage?

In sorting through these questions, policymakers face both managerial and policy dilemmas. Making the system user friendly—for instance, deciding eligibility case by case—risks making reform too expensive. Keeping costs down risks making the system more rule bound. Collecting subsidies, channeling them to health providers, controlling costs, and serving the poor is no mean feat. Ensuring that the money gets to where it is needed will require highly skilled management.

Competing Approaches

Health care reform is not a choice between relying on government or the private sector. Nor is it a choice between easy or complex administration. All health care reform will be administratively complex. The choice, rather, is this: which kind of program do Americans prefer? Approaches that rely more on government authority invite contentions that private autonomy is being compromised. Approaches that rely more on private markets raise issues of whether public goals such as universal coverage are being met. America cannot in any case escape hard choices. So making the choices will require careful assessment of the management burdens that each option imposes and thoughtful reflection on how those burdens can be managed to produce the desired results.

Every state is now wrestling with health care reform on its own, with varying success. The seven states that the National Commission on the State and Local Public Service studied have used different management approaches in different ways. Each state is looking for the best administrative approaches, but each has adapted them in very different ways to meet local needs, political climates, and administrative structures. In coping with the burdens of national health care reform, some states have come a long way, while others will need substantial technical assistance and, perhaps, money to devise the structures, hire experienced managers, and otherwise build the capacity to implement health care reform. If national health care reform requires skillful management of implementing strategies, it also requires that the administrative diversity of the states be taken fully into account (table 1-3).

The lesson: the choice is not whether to have a government role in ensuring health care, but what kind of role to have. That choice requires focusing on problems of implementation and the limits of federalism. How we choose will lead us to rely more on some strategies, less on others. But the ability to manage these tools, especially in the states, varies widely. Making health care reform work will require building the needed capacity and defining the functions of the different participants.

Defining Federal and State Roles

Defining federal and state health care roles has to begin with the most important health alliance of all, federalism. Health care reform promises to be the most important event involving federalism in a generation. If it is to work, Washington and the states will have important functions to perform. To perform well, each will have to be clear on what its function is. There needs to be a sensible division of labor that plays to the strengths of American federalism: establishing broad national policy while allowing the states to match that policy to special local conditions. At the same time, the cacophony and conflict that have marked past intergovernmental efforts must be avoided.[9]

The Federal Role

To strike the balance of federalism, the federal government must define the basic rules of the health care plan and ensure that the plan can be carried out successfully.

The first and most important function is to define precisely who and what health care reform will encompass. Will it guarantee coverage to all Americans or simply guarantee that they will be able to purchase coverage? Will it adequately pay for health care for the old and the poor? Will it prevent gaps in coverage caused by preexisting conditions or moves between employers with different health plans? Health care reform will require the federal government, in particular, to determine those parameters that are of national concern and must be uniform in application and those matters in which other goals, especially responsiveness to state-by-state variations, are more important.

In practice, establishing the limits of the plan means defining the basic benefits to which citizens will be entitled. Benefits must be allocated between emergency and preventive care and among medical, surgical, mental health, dental, and pharmaceutical coverage. Everyone agrees that "medically necessary" procedures ought to be covered. Almost no one agrees on what that means. Health care reform will require the federal government to put flesh on the bones of health care reform by defining what will be covered.

The federal government must also decide how to finance the system. Will government itself pay? And if so, should it be the federal government or the state governments? How much of the cost should employers pay, and what should employees be responsible for? Even if the federal government does not itself pay for the system, it must clearly and fairly determine who will.

In any plan the federal government will have to measure what it has wrought. The system will be complex; managing that complexity will require a system that roots out and solves problems as quickly as possible. The government can promote such action only if it can track the results—in quality delivered, ease and equity of access, and price. Health care reform will require the federal government to ensure that the terms of the entitlement are met.

Finally, the federal government has a responsibility to the integrity of the health care reform process. It must determine who participates in decisionmaking and who makes final decisions. When national decisions are made, will the federal government ensure that the state governments are represented in the process? Will governors or their representatives have a seat on a national health board? How much decisionmaking power will the federal government share with the states and its other partners? The federal government must not only do good, but it must be seen to do good.

Health care reform will require the federal government to determine rules and structures in which everyone can have confidence. The most difficult part of building such confidence will be moving to a more uniform system of health coverage on the foundation of such different state capacities and structures. The federal government will have to plan the transition carefully. It will have to be ready with technical assistance and perhaps financial support for less experienced states. Most impor-

Table 1-3. Health Care Reform Management Techniques Used in Seven States

Management technique	Minnesota	Washington State	California	Florida	New York	Mississippi	Texas
Regulation	Minnesota Health Care Commission designed the plan, which was enacted by the state legislature. Regulation is within the Minnesota Department of Health.	Health Services Commission charged with designing a uniform benefits package, determining maximum premium level. Inflation reduction specified in statute.	Market reforms for small business firms' (5-50) health insurance include guaranteed issuance, renewability, and portability of all products. Limits exclusions on preexisting conditions to six months.	In 1995 state will require employers to provide insurance or pay into a state insurance fund if voluntary subscription is low.	State requires small business firms' (3-50 employees) plans to be community rated.		
Institution building	Integrated service networks of state providers arrange or deliver health services for a fixed price; may be nonprofits or cooperatives. Volunteer pooling arrangements.	Four regional noncompeting voluntary health insurance purchasing cooperatives must serve at least 150,000 people, allow any person or group to participate, and offer every plan available in the region.	Health Insurance Plan of California available to small businesses (5-50 employees) regardless of group health status. Small employer group purchasing pool established.	Eleven state-chartered, voluntary, nonprofit community health purchasing alliances available to small businesses (up to 50 employees), uninsured residents, state employees, and medicaid recipients.	State encourages development of regional health networks.	Virtually no managed-care structures (HMOs, PPOs); shortage of primary care doctors. Health Department has begun to establish informal networks between local community health organizations and doctors, both primary care and specialists.	Texas insurance purchasing alliance: statewide, nonprofit purchasing cooperative for small companies (3-50 employees). Voluntary business-run purchasing alliances allowed for small businesses.

	Information gathering	Subsidies
	Health Care Commission charged with working toward universal coverage by 1997.	Minnesota Care offers coverage to uninsured low-income families with children and individuals with incomes up to 275 percent of poverty. Enrollees contribute to premiums based on income.
	Health Services Commission will monitor participation and spending.	Basic health plan offers benefits to uninsured low-income (up to 200 percent of poverty) with premiums based on income.
	Community health purchasing alliances rate health care providers, collect proposals for basic and extended coverage options, calculate best prices and services, and provide members with comparative information on available plans.	Major Risk Medical Insurance Program and Access for Infants and Mothers (AIM) offer subsidization for low-income and uninsured.
	State Board of Quality Improvements will identify and evaluate quality and efficacy of state medical practices.	Child Health Insurance Plan: subsidized program for low-income children.
	Governor's Commission on Health Care developing initial strategies for access, delivery, and financing.	
	Governor, Lt. Governor, and Speaker had task force in 1992. State Legislative Budget Office charged with developing options for state reform.	

tant, it will have to establish a reasonable and predictable division of labor between the federal and the state governments.

The State Role

Under most plans the state governments will be on the front lines of implementation. They are likely to have the responsibility for delivering the results, which defines their basic functions.

In most plans, state governments will link the governmental apparatus with for-profit and nonprofit health care providers. If health care reform resembles the creation of huge shopping malls, state governments will be the malls' developers and managers. They will determine who gets to open health care stores, how the stores will offer their services, and how customers may shop. They will also be responsible for ensuring the quality of the care customers receive. Reform will also require the states to construct and oversee the health marketplace, to develop pooled purchasing or other organizational arrangements, and ensure that they work productively.

All the plans will create heavy demands for building institutions. In some plans the states will have to create alliances or other cooperative purchasing plans. In others they will need a far stronger capacity to regulate and oversee the private health market. Reform will require state officials to become skillful institution builders and even more skilled managers to produce success.

These tasks will require states to collect and analyze massive amounts of data. Many of the management problems of the status quo stem from inadequate information and insufficient ability to follow through on the problems the information identifies. State governments must be able to discover problems while they are still small. The states will also typically be responsible for collecting the raw data on which federal decisions rest. Health care reform will require the states to become skilled data managers.

The primary reason for relying on federalism to begin with is to ensure that the system is responsive to citizens. To guarantee responsiveness, however, the states will have to redefine their job of representing citizens' interests. The states have always been challenged in representing their citizens. With health care reform they will have daunting new challenges in making the system responsive. They will have to work with new organizational arrangements, through new administrative challenges, and in partnership with new public-private hybrids to incorporate responsiveness to the public interest into the competition of the private marketplace.

Determining the roles comes down to this. The federal government must define the national interest and the state governments' role in contributing to that interest. It must create the right incentives for the states to fulfill their responsibilities. And it must assess the system's ability to achieve those results.

If the federal government's role is to design the basic system, the states are likely to be responsible for health care reform's internal wiring. They will have to build the institutions and oversee the mechanisms that actually deliver care. Most important, they will have to ensure that the broad policy goals reflect citizens' needs.

The lesson: health care reform assigns different roles to the federal and state governments. Understanding those roles, and building the capacity to meet them, is the precondition for successful reform.

The Phasing of Transition

Making health care reform work requires identifying and solving the critical problems on which success depends. Any plan will be complex. But managing that complexity demands understanding which steps must be taken first and which should come later. It also requires avoiding those things that cannot be done at all. And the very different state capacities must be taken into account in working toward a national solution. Finally, it requires great skill in managing the transition from the status quo to the new system to ensure public confidence.

Do First Things First

In any reform plan as complex as health care reform will be, it is impossible to do everything at once. In a reform built on such a varied base of capacity in the states and among for-profit and nonprofit partners, to seek quick uniformity would be a disaster. Success, rather, depends critically on defining first principles and first steps.

A commitment to any policy change must begin by making the health care system more user friendly. It must be designed, from the top down, to serve the needs of citizens effectively. The problem, of course, is that citizens' desires often exceed their willingness to pay for satisfying those desires. What can health reform afford to give them? How can it manage the inevitable trade-offs? Government will be a crucial gatekeeper in the system: in balancing cost and service, guaranteeing access and quality, and fitting together the system's diverse administrative elements to ensure that citizens' needs are not ignored.

The next most important step is for the federal government to make clear the functions of participants. Assigning the roles makes clear not only who is accountable to whom for what but also the process used to produce accountability. Rules on access and subsidies, for instance, must be uniform and should be the province of the federal government. Matters that need to take account of local conditions should be the province of the state governments. Choice among service providers and other matters that can be resolved by competition among health providers can be left to the for-profit and nonprofit sectors.

After roles are delineated, the rules can be developed. With so many participants at so many levels involved in health policy, setting the rules defines the relationships among them. Everyone from federal officials supervising the system through state officials in critical intermediate positions to private health care providers needs to have a predictable base on which to build the new relationships. Delineating regulations will define these relationships.

Although regulation will fix the relationships, implementation will require creating whole new kinds of institutions or making dramatic changes in existing ones. Health care reform can press ahead without stopping to build the institutions first. But it will work far better, especially for its customers, if the institutions are built early in the process.

Supplying financing, whether through tax incentives or subsidies, can come next. Money is the engine that drives health care, as it does all other government systems. Establishing the channels along which it will flow will ensure that it most easily gets to where it is needed.

Finally, most of the health care reform plans anticipate that managers will need to collect information about the quality of the service provided. Constructing this system is the last step in the chain. Some feedback will be simple: there is evidence that word-of-mouth reputations of physicians and hospitals conditions a great many health care choices. Still, with so much political involvement in debating various plans and so much money at issue, it is impossible that health care reform will escape more quantifiable political and managerial scrutiny. Careful analysis of results will be important so that elected officials and public managers know what they have created and how to improve what is not working well. Because it is important that the system produce such information, it will be important that the capacity for information collection be designed in from the beginning. Results will shape the perceptions and public support for reform. Even if it is the last step in the process, information is critical to reform's long-term success.

Some might argue that these steps ought to be initiated in a different order. Indeed, in most building projects, some pieces can be added in any order. But there is no denying two inescapable considerations. First, some pieces must come first. A roof cannot be nailed down unless the foundation is dug first and the framing constructed. In health care reform, putting service to recipients first is the foundation. Defining the roles and setting the rules ought to precede building the institutions and supplying the money.

The second consideration is that careful preliminary consideration of the order in which reforms will be implemented is far better than pressing blindly ahead. Without careful thought the reform effort risks trying to do everything at once or doing the wrong things first. Either course is likely to aggravate the partners (federal and state; for-profit and nonprofit) in service provision. Either will drive up costs, increase delays, reduce quality, and disappoint service recipients.

Most of the national health care reform debate has swirled around who will pay and what benefits citizens will receive. Cutting through these concerns to the management issues is not easy. But the more planners succeed in doing that before legislation is passed, the greater the chances of producing real and sustained success.

Limit Reform to the Doable

Not only must policymakers do the most important things first, they must not try to do things that cannot be done. All the plans presuppose information and institutions that may simply be beyond the reach of administrative technologies. Here are a few illustrations from a sample of three plans.

The Health Security Act would create new challenges and hurdles administratively even for those states aggressively moving forward with reform. But this is only the beginning. The Clinton plan envisions the establishment of a fifteen-member national quality management council that would develop dozens of national performance measures to be used to evaluate every health provider system in terms of accessibility, appropriateness of services, outcomes of services and procedures, prevention of diseases, and much more. The act goes into great detail about the consumer surveys to be conducted to assess quality plan by plan and state by state. Information from these surveys and other research would result in annual report cards on plans.

But developing a report card that captures the quality of a plan and will be meaningful to consumers is not feasible very soon. Not a single state now has a data-based management system approaching what would be necessary to conduct such performance reviews. And even if the information technology and procedural hurdles could be cleared, the intellectual ones would prove daunting. Scientific understanding depends on the ability to identify relevant variables, specify how they relate one to another, and determine how (if at all) the relationships among them can be measured and tested. A national quality management council presupposes a level of scientific understanding about the causal links among medical interventions, population characteristics, and health outcomes that neither the states nor the federal government possesses.

The Managed Competition Act, proposed by Representatives Jim Cooper of Tennessee and Fred Grandy of Iowa, would establish health plan purchasing cooperatives (HPPCs) that would contract with accountable health plans (AHPs).[10] The cooperatives could include an entire state or one or more metropolitan statistical areas, containing at least 250,000 persons, within a state. Initially, governors would appoint HPPC boards. A national health care standards commission would oversee the plans, which would be required to provide a uniform set of benefits.

One administrative hurdle here is that the IRS would be responsible for tracking individual and corporate deductible levels and ensuring their accuracy on tax returns. And, of course, the IRS has had trouble managing the existing tax-processing system. If each state established only one cooperative, there would be at least 600 different individual deductibles (one HPPC times the act's four enrollment classes times three age brackets times fifty states). Most states, however, would establish multiple HPPCs, so the IRS would have to take cognizance of hundreds of HPPC boundaries and thousands of different deductibles. People living around the corner from one another could be subject to different requirements. It is impossible to imagine that taxpayers could cope with the complicated tax schedules or that the IRS could effectively manage them.

The plan is virtually silent about the role of the states. But the implementation of many provisions—the authorization, licensing, and oversight of AHPs; assistance for individuals and families with incomes below 200 percent of their state's poverty line; paperwork reduction and simplification protocols—will fall to the states. The act does not specify what, if any, financial or other incentives the states will have to shoulder these heavy administrative burdens.

The Consumer Choice Health Security Act, proposed by Senator Don Nickles of Oklahoma, guarantees all Americans access to insurance that is portable and available without regard to preexisting conditions.[11] It is modeled after the Federal Employee Health Benefit program. The act would replace tax exclusions for employer-sponsored health plans with individual tax credits. For every $100 spent on health insurance premiums, or contributed to a medical savings account, or spent on out-of-pocket medical expenses, an individual or family would pay $25 less in taxes. The secretary of the Department of Health and Human Services would require all health care providers to submit claims to health insurance companies in accordance with federal standards, while the attorney general would establish a program to exempt certain providers from antitrust laws relating to the delivery of health care services.

Although this act is often discussed as one of several incremental reform proposals, there is nothing incremental about its administrative requirements. The tax credits would take effect on January 1, 1997. Thus within fewer than three years the secretary of Health and Human Services would need to specify the standards for qualified health plans and establish the regulatory machinery necessary to certify plans if the states, under penalty of a loss of federal dollars, failed to do so. Moreover, the act would preempt state laws pertaining to mandated benefits and services and require states to standardize and streamline their processing of health insurance claims. The act says nothing about precisely how this is to be achieved.

Managing the Transition

The transition to health care reform will not be easy. Cynics can hide behind that warning to oppose any change at all. That cynicism, however, must be met with three observations. First, the status quo itself is full of dangerous uncertainty for many Americans: the risk of developing an illness that will not be covered, of changing jobs and discovering that preexisting conditions are excluded from the new employer's health insurance plan, of having insurance canceled or its costs escalate beyond affordability. The uncertainties of health care reform dim when compared with the risks of the status quo.

Second, even if reform produces a more complex system, there can be large returns from administrative complexity. More complexity may be justified if it can reduce uncertainties about health care insurance and increase confidence in the quality and affordability of care. One need not only compare the complexity of reform with the complexity of the status quo. One also needs to weigh the improvement in coverage and care that added complexity may buy.

Finally, a system's complexity is less important than its usability. Complex systems can be more user friendly than simple ones if they are designed well. Banks have developed extremely sophisticated electronic systems to allow their customers to withdraw cash and deposit checks at machines around the community at any hour of the day and night. These systems are not simple, but their complexity does not matter because they are user friendly and they work.

In thinking about complexity, therefore, one needs to think about the returns from added complexity. Engineering complexity so that it does not become a barrier to service must also be considered. Indeed, citizens' confidence in what they will receive from health care reform is a critical element for building political support. And it certainly will be a prerequisite for continued support of any reform system that the federal government creates.

The lesson: reform must build on a solid foundation, with the critical steps taken first. Those steps that cannot be achieved should not be attempted. And all of the steps have to make the system as user friendly for citizens as is possible. Careful management will minimize the transition costs. These three steps taken together will determine the ultimate success of health care reform.

Conclusion: Reform Can Work

Lost in the debate over competing health care reform plans is the consensus that reform is essential. Rarely in American history has such a consensus emerged so quickly. Policymakers have rapidly moved from whether reform is needed to what it should look like. Our fundamental argument in this volume is that the "what" has to be answered in the context of the how it can be managed. Health care reform can work, but only if policymakers work hard to build in success from the beginning.

Much depends on how federal policymakers choose to lead. If the drive to pass some legislation—any legislation—swamps the difficult search for a reform package that can gain political support and work administratively, there can be little cause for hope. But if policymakers assess the problems of implementation, management, and federalism before passing a reform plan, chances for success will vastly increase and a new chapter in America's history of governance will be written.

Any conceivable national health care reform will be trying to do things—in scope, scale, and time—far beyond any domestic policy initiative the United States has ever attempted. Never before has it tried to reform such a huge piece of the economy. And it has never attempted, since mobilization to fight World War II, to produce such a big change in such a short period of time. If reform is not managed carefully, and if management success is not built into the design of the policy, reform will surely court disaster. America cannot afford to punish the sick or make the healthy ill through ambitious reform that not only falls short of its promises but creates new and unforeseen problems. The more policymakers pay attention, from the beginning, to the management issues of health care reform, the better results will be.

2 ‖ Health Alliances: Functions, Forms, and Federalism

James R. Tallon, Jr., and
Lawrence D. Brown

ONCE A significant national health care reform program becomes law, the spotlight will turn to the fifty states, in each of which officials will be asking the classic implementation question, "What do we do now?" The way they answer that question will determine much of the success of a new national policy.

Different reform strategies pose distinct managerial challenges, and the states will tackle their tasks with due regard for their particular traditions and tastes. Generic administrative advice is cheap indeed. Nonetheless, it may be useful to anticipate and analyze the administrative tasks that are likely to loom large across a range of reform options. Such an exercise may contribute, at least marginally, to states' managerial preparedness, to a better understanding by political leaders of what they might do to make reform work, and to fuller public deliberations on matching means to ends. We examine here some administrative challenges of implementing health alliances in the states. Alliances figure prominently in President Bill Clinton's reform proposal, but, more to the point, they crystallize many issues that arise in most reform plans that stand a chance of enactment by the federal government or the states.

The Rationale for Alliances

Most nations with universal health care coverage take pains to hold payers (insurance organizations) accountable to purchasers (those who put up the money for health care coverage).[1] The U.S. system is peculiar in that payers largely emerged as creatures of providers (physicians, hospitals) and have served providers' interests more often than those of purchasers. This legacy is especially hard on purchasers such as small businesses and individuals, which offer up few "lives" to the insurance market and therefore exert limited leverage in bargaining for favorable rates and reasonable terms.[2] The problem is especially critical for the 39 million or so Americans who have no medical insurance, for most of them are workers, mainly in small firms, or dependents of workers.

If policymakers decline to adopt a single-payer system or some other model in which government insures the whole citizenry, they need mechanisms to correct these market imperfections. Insurance reforms (such as community rating or guaranteed issue) go part of the way but do not, some contend, offer a satisfactory solution. Something more may be needed to perform functions indispensable to a successful refashioning of insurance markets that are now badly broken. The most widely embraced answer is the regional health alliance, apparently first fleshed out by Alain Enthoven (who made the case for health insurance purchasing cooperatives), and then adopted by the Jackson Hole group and the Clinton administration, which devised the current moniker.[3]

For various reasons (noted below), alliances have proved to be a controversial innovation and may or may not make their way into national legislation. If they are adopted, in any form, the states will doubtless have a major role in setting them up and making them work. But even if they fall by the political wayside, the states will still be obliged to find other ways of performing the functions assigned to alliances. In this chapter we explore some practical issues that arise in moving alliances from theory into institutional reality, with special attention to the roles the states will probably play as decisionmakers and mediators between the central government and the regions.

Functions and Frictions

The basic rationale for alliances, or for some comparable entity, is that effective reform of U.S. health insurance markets requires that certain tasks or functions be performed and that some competent organization, new or existing, tackle them. Three core functions are probably fundamental to achieving affordable universal coverage (at least by means short of a single-payer strategy). Three others may not be generic but are still key to most versions of managed competition.

Concert Purchaser Leverage

If universal coverage is to be affordable, U.S. policymakers must find ways to put providers under tighter fiscal control. If market forces are the chosen instrument, some means must be found to make payers take account of purchasers' preferences. Health alliances would do this because they would represent blocks of insurance buyers and drive hard bargains with payers (insurers or health plans) that could compete effectively only if they disciplined the providers in their networks.

Beyond this boilerplate image of alliances, deep disputes arise between those who want alliances to *influence* markets (rather as farmers' cooperatives would) and those who would have them *reorganize* markets by the exercise of enormous, perhaps near-monopsony, power. How large should or must alliances be? The Clinton administration would require that all employers with 5,000 or fewer workers join the alliances established in their region. Larger employers would constitute their own alliances.[4] Their argument is that smaller alliances would suffer adverse selection (risk pooling would be attractive mainly to poorer risks while healthier types shopped elsewhere for better bargains), would wield too little clout to shape and steer the market, and would be unable to spread the costs of expensive populations such as medicaid recipients in a single-tiered system of coverage. Critics counter that such mammoths replace the original notion of a farmers' cooperative, setting up amidst a range of more or less organized purchasing bodies, with government-sponsored bureaucracies that stifle true competition. They believe that alliances should serve much smaller businesses, up to a maximum of, say, 1,000, 100, or even 50 workers.

Supporters of alliances also divide over whether they should be mandatory or voluntary for the groups (of whatever size) they would serve. The administration contends that membership must be obligatory lest adverse selection defeat true pooling and spreading of risks and drive up alliance members' costs. Federal legislation requiring that most employers join and finance these new and untested entities is a hard pill to swallow, however, and some analysts urge that alliances be deployed and tested on a voluntary basis, that is, as a potential source of good deals for those who want to use them.

Should regions be allowed to sustain competing health alliances? Those, like the Clinton planners, who oppose this option contend that competing alliances would lose economies of scale in purchasing, stretch the ranks of talented staff too thin, increase bureaucracy and duplication, encourage cost shifting among plans, and, most serious, invite adverse selection as purchasers scramble to sign up where risks and costs are lowest. Others think that the logic of competition obviously justifies choices that let buyers go wherever they can get the best terms for health insurance.

In resolving these disagreements, federal policymakers have three main options. First, they can devise a uniform national blueprint that the states must try to implement. (Under the Clinton plan, states could adopt a single-payer system or one based on health alliances, which could be nonprofit organizations or agencies of the state governments.) Second, they can permit states to answer these questions for themselves, at least within limits. Or, third, they can decline to enshrine alliances in a national plan and let states decide whether they want to create them and, if so, in what form. Each correlative course of action—implementing a detailed federal vision of alliances, deciding how to define alliances, and working to concert purchaser leverage without alliances—throws challenges to the states.

Avert Preferred Risk Selection

According to the Clinton planners, some new entity—namely, alliances—must assume the function of enrolling individuals and families in insurance plans. The task cannot be left to insurers, who will cherrypick better risks "as surely as water rolls downhill."[5] Not everyone concurs. Some would adopt and implement the basics of insurance reform—such as guaranteed issue, portability, limits on exclusion of coverage for preexisting conditions, and community rating—and see if experience suggests that alliances are needed.[6] Others believe that community rating renders alliances superfluous.[7] Unless large mandatory alliances are established across the nation by federal fiat, the states will have to invent their own mechanisms to prevent preferred-risk selection by insurers—a task for which their previous ventures in insurance regulation hardly begin to prepare them.

Even if alliances are deemed necessary to preventing cherrypicking, they might not be sufficient. Health plans may try to discourage high users from signing on by, for example, keeping the number of high-cost specialty services few and remote. Everyone's favorite corrective is risk-adjusted payments to plans that enroll disproportionate numbers of high users; these remove the financial spur to discrimination. If alliances administer the risk adjustments, states will need to oversee their work. Without alliances, the states themselves will presumably implement both insurance reform and the risk adjustments (or some functional substitute) that ensure true universality of coverage.

Empower and Inform Consumers

If universal coverage and cost containment are to be harmonized, consumers must be sensitive to and informed about value for money in health care. They must carefully consider costs as they shop for the levels of access and quality they want. But how are they to know? The Clinton plan expects health alliances to act as neutral brokers, gathering and analyzing data on plan performance, encoding it in report cards, transmitting the information to consumers, and perhaps helping them to interpret it. Skeptics contend that this vision asks too much of the alliances, the data, and the consumers. The data that tell consumers everything they might ever want to know about plan behavior are not now available and will be slow to develop, and their interpretation generates disputes even among experts. But whether one envisions a large-scale quest for comprehensive data and analysis or a slowly building elucidation of select aspects of the system, the states have their work cut out for them. If health alliances take the lead, the states must see that they do it right. If alliances do not or cannot perform this role, states will have to decide how far, and how, to take it on.

Administer and Disburse Subsidies

If the costs of coverage are to be met in part by a combination of employer and worker contributions, questions arise about ability to pay. Many smaller and less profitable firms insist that neither they nor their typically lower-wage employees can shoulder 80 percent and 20 percent, respectively, of the cost of a basic benefits package. The Clinton team sought to ease their anxieties by proposing that the total contribution of smaller firms be capped at a low percentage of payroll and that the neediest get federal subsidies to help meet their costs. Many economists contend, however, that business itself does not, and would not, bear these costs but rather would transfer them to workers as trade-offs against wage growth. If so, the workers, who ultimately bear the costs of coverage, should get the subsidies. And of course, some hybrid approach is not only possible but likely. However one designs the subsidy scheme, there must be an administrative device to verify the eligibility of firms and workers for subsidies and to disburse these sums. The Clinton plan assigns these tasks to the alliances. Or a state agency could perform these roles directly, although few have much experience in doing so.[8]

Collect and Allocate Premiums

An employer-based strategy obviously means that employers pay much of the cost of covering their workers. Firms could continue to perform this function as they do now, but the Clinton plan would end employers' direct role in choosing workers' plans, so individuals and households would belong to alliances that enroll their members in the health plans those members choose. Alliances could presumably instruct employers whom to pay, but administrative efficiency argues that employers should pay alliances that in turn pay to the plans premiums appropriately adjusted to the risks of enrollees. This role of fiscal conduit looks straightforward enough on paper, but in practice it channels many billions of premium dollars into (and, one hopes, through) the hands of new and perhaps thinly staffed novice organizations. States must be vigilant about fiscal probity and accounting. If alliances fail to be enacted, however, states must enforce mandates (that is, assure timely and full employer and employee contributions to premiums) in a universal system.

Negotiate and Persuade

The Clinton plan hopes to give every American stable, secure health coverage while steering the rate of growth of health costs down to the rate of growth of the consumer price index within a few years. These goals can be met simultaneously only if health plans agree to cover everyone while enforcing internal efficiencies that generate premiums low enough to meet the cost targets. The plan recommends a regulatory "backstop"—regional caps on the allowable rate of increase of insurance premiums—if market forces fail, but the rosy scenario is that the interplay of purchaser specifications, articulated by the alliances, and provider adaptations, mediated by plans bidding for business, will do the job. Although the Clinton plan gives alliances no formal negotiating roles or powers, if such market forces are to work, alliances will probably have to negotiate with the plans and exert pressure about both the premiums they charge and the access and quality of care the premiums buy. These roles imply, in turn, that alliances will have extensive knowledge and strong backbones, and that states will identify and move to repair alliances that prove to be deficient in these respects.

The central dilemma for federal and state policymakers is whether alliances are necessary or sufficient to perform these six functions. Granted that a system dedicated to disciplined market dynamics must somehow meet these functions, what is one to conclude about the alliance construct? One school of thought argues that those who think carefully through the requisites of these tasks return, however grudgingly, to the Clinton blueprint; nothing less works. Others contend that these tasks can be handled well enough by alliances far smaller and weaker than those Clinton proposes, and still others think that it makes more sense to build capacity within established state agencies than it does to entrust these multiple and complex duties to a new national system of untested alliances at an artificial (regional) level of (quasi) government. However these disputes may get resolved in Washington, for the states there is no exit: either they will oversee and supervise alliances' efforts to perform these roles, or they will tackle all (or many) of them themselves.

Implementing Alliances

Health alliances are often described as the linchpin of the Clinton scheme, and the states are the linchpins of a workable alliance system. The Clinton plan would have each state submit to a national health board its plans for organizing the system; establish one or more alliances for defined regions; ensure that families in each alliance have a choice of health plans; see to it that families get the subsidies to which they are entitled; set capital rules for health plans; devise standards for the financial reporting, reserves, and auditing of health plans; certify plans along a range of criteria; create and guarantee funds to cover the obligations of health plans that fail; secure continuous coverage for enrollees in defunct plans; assure that regional alliances collect the monies owed them; help alliances determine eligibility for subsidies and cost-sharing sums; and pay (in part) for medicaid enrollees in alliances.[9] This weighty job description poses three broad types of implementation challenges: structure and governance, knowledge and capacity, and external relations.

Structure and Governance

Under the Clinton program, states have a large say in deciding the organizational structure of the alliances and how they will be run. Three issues will be especially difficult. First, states are to determine the number of health alliances within their boundaries (alliances cannot cross state lines). How the lines are drawn will establish the distribution of risks, use, and costs within each region and thus the premium costs alliance members will pay. Firms are likely to apply considerable pressure to draw lines that reduce their costs, yet obviously each member cannot expect to have exclusively low-cost compatriots, so these decisions may, as the director of medicaid in Texas put it, take on the character of "public school finance meets legislative redistricting."[10]

Second, states will decide the administrative structure of the alliances within a federal menu that currently has three main options. A state can choose a single-payer system, but presumably few will elect to do so, at least at first. They can make alliances state agencies, but one wonders if many businesses—the prime constituents of the new entities—will favor this mode of representation. Or they can be nonprofit agencies run by boards with equal numbers of employers and consumers.

What governance structure makes sense?[11] Employers and consumers are not homogeneous categories. How much, and how, should blocs within each camp be represented? These boards will direct the flow of billions of dollars and influence the health care of millions of citizens. Ideology, partisanship, and the jealousy and distrust that go with them will inevitably enter in, which could generate pressure for direct election. Should the boards be appointed, perhaps by governors, from lists compiled by business and consumer groups? Does this scheme give established organizations undue power? Which groups, in a sometimes crowded organizational field, should be included? Moreover, unlike the nonprofit, multimember health systems agencies (HSAs) of the 1970s and 1980s, alliances will have major operational duties. Board posts will not be merely honorific, and the tasks at hand will demand substantial investments of time by people bringing significant expertise. Will the right people be available, and on what terms? What works in one state may be all wrong for another. But, given congressional anxieties about entrusting major new powers to the wrong partisan hands, will legislation leave states the flexibility they need to organize these new structures to fit their preferences?

Knowledge and Capacity

Once alliances are established, who will run them day to day? Will they know what they are doing? How do states prepare for the challenges of staffing? We noted above the complexities of assuring boards with adequate commitment and expertise; similar questions arise for staff. Should these be political or civil service jobs? (Each has its pros and cons.) People with experience in insurance and employee benefits may be numerous and savvy enough to staff them adequately, but how much must alliances pay to secure their services?

Prescriptions for staffing should be drawn in light of the alliances' task structure: what are they expected to do? States certify health plans, but alliances join them in monitoring plan performance across a range of variables. Alliances will, among other duties, assure the adequacy of the plans' services, facilities, and staff; issue report cards that inform consumers about quality of care; collect and disburse insurance premium payments; and determine eligibility for subsidies and pay them. The Congressional Budget Office noted that alliances "would combine the functions of purchasing agents, contract negotiators, welfare agencies, financial intermediaries, collectors of premiums, developers and managers of information systems, and coordinators of the flow of information and money between themselves and other alliances."[12] The CBO observes further that to do their work the alliances will need "extensive management information systems and access to national information networks," plus the capacity to conduct or contract for surveys and data analyses. Their jobs would require "collecting, maintaining, and updating large amounts of information on individuals, employers, and health plans," in order to track enrollment and nonenrollment in plans according to the risk characteristics of members and whether members are clients of public programs; determining the eligibility of employers and families for premium subsidies; assessing eligibility for reductions in cost sharing; tracking cost-sharing payments by low-income people in high-cost-sharing plans; and monitoring the premiums families owe, with due regard to their hours of employment and changes in family status.[13]

Risk management is but one sobering illustration of the complexity of some of these tasks. If alliances cannot assess the incidence and costs of risk prospectively with much success—and experts agree that available indicators predict quite poorly—then it is hard to deter preferred-risk selection by promising plans that they will be fairly compensated for accepting riskier enrollees. Alliances can evaluate risk and cost retroactively and make payments accordingly, but that approach has problems of its own. It is not easy to disentangle the effects of health status risks from the consequences of management practices in health plans, and there should be no reward for laxness on the latter count. Moreover, retrospective payment interferes with the incentives supposedly inherent in managed care to accept risk and organize care efficiently in order to remain within fixed budgets set in advance.

The many demands on alliances' knowledge and skill would be substantial in all states, highly onerous in many, and (at least initially) downright indecipherable in some. ("We are at zero when it comes to expertise," lamented a health official in one Deep South state.) If these jobs are tackled unobtrusively and with few staff ("nonbureaucratically"), they may be done superficially and poorly. But can they be done usefully and well without sizable staffs, big budgets, or stacks of data, in short, without a major bureaucratic production? The larger the alliances (the higher the cutoff figure for mandatory membership), the more salient these questions become.

A closely related unknown is whether alliance staffs will have the organizational technologies they need to do their work. Their multiple tasks would seem to argue for multitalented staffers, who may not be in abundant supply. A top public administrator and veteran of years of debate on health care reform in Washington State argues that one needs "people who know the health care delivery system, people who understand risk and insurance, and people who understand state government, government programs, in the political process."[14] Because political leaders have labored to assure both the general and special publics that alliances will not be "another layer of government bureaucracy," but rather will be spartan entities thinly staffed by facilitators, it is questionable that alliances will be well equipped to demand, let alone to find, a stable supply of the numbers and types of staffers they will need. The larger the number of alliances within and across the states, the harder it will be to staff them all properly, which would seem to counsel against the temptation to award each politically cohesive and vocal community its own alliance.

External Relations

The complexities of implementing health alliances do not end with their internal structures and capacities. Because they are the focal institution asked to pull together an otherwise fragmented and unaccountable system, alliances will deal with many groups whose behavior they must seek to influence and who will pressure them in turn. Some examples follow.

BUSINESS. Although some theorists view alliances as a belated answer to the U.S. business community's prayers and dreams—at last, an institutional mechanism to put the purchaser in the driver's seat— major business organizations have reacted cautiously to this policy innovation. Handwringing over health costs notwithstanding, many firms are reluctant to sever the link between employment status and choice of health plan: some because they want to continue to run and fine-tune plans that they think work well, others because they do not want to pay 80 percent of an alliancewide average premium to a new entity and then lose voice about where the money goes. Still others distrust on principle new government-sponsored agencies that stand largely immune from the competitive dynamics that business reflexively endorses, and yet another camp doubts that alliances will effectively curb the growth of health insurance premiums, of which the federal government would now compel business to pay the lion's share. In business, then, alliances find not a natural, newly activated, and grateful constituency, but rather a continuum of opinion dominated by skeptics who remain to be convinced that alliances will serve their interests well.

Alliances may have a hard time pleasing this critical crowd. They will collect contributions (mandatory under the Clinton plan) from employers, some of whom will be contributing (involuntarily) for the first time or paying more (80 percent of premiums) for workers' coverage than previously. They will allocate premium funds among health plans, interpret legal criteria for subsidies, and award the subsidies. The alliances will need to ensure accuracy of bookkeeping, reasonableness of documentation burdens, honest handling of funds, veracity of employer statements about profits, and timeliness in responding to business queries. If these functions are performed poorly or slowly, the alliance boards—and presumably their state and federal overseers—may be inundated with complaints from the purchaser interests most directly and intensely affected by their doings.

CONSUMERS. The Clinton plan builds on the existing system by retaining employers' contributions to workers' coverage, but also departs from it radically by ending the employers' role in choosing plans for workers. The alliances will construct the menu and present it directly to consumers, who will choose for themselves. Lest households be overwhelmed by the representations of competing plans about cost, quality, and access, not to mention the trade-offs they offer among these variables, alliances must work to "empower" consumers in a newly dynamic marketplace. This job implies presenting data that are germane to consumer concerns and clearly understandable. Deciding what data are truly useful in decisionmaking, and knowing when enough is enough, are not easy judgments. Hundreds of pages recounting multiple measures of columns of indicators for dozens of plans presumably go too far; on the other hand, a little knowledge may be a dangerous thing.

Nor will the data, however statistically significant and artfully edited, always be clear on their face. Alliances may need to interpret data and dispel confusion. In Washington State, alliances are, among other things, "health benefits experts" offering employers and consumers a "cost effective place to go to have their questions answered about quality of care, plan changes, network stability, benefits, [and] cost."[15] This counseling role, however, has rather nebulous staffing and legal connotations. The states are not well prepared to help alliances tackle these tasks or to ensure that they are performing them reliably. Few states, for instance, house health staff thoroughly versed in the art and science of quality monitoring, still less in synthesizing the features of a range of plans into report cards that invite consumers to make invidious distinctions among them. If alliances and their state overseers fail as traffic cops, the combination of competing plans and confused consumers could spell chaos.

Moreover, mere ordinary confusion will doubtless suffice to incite the litigation to which disconsolate Americans cheerfully resort. The more integrated the contractual arrangements and organizational links among purchasers, providers, and payers, the more extensive and murky are the potential chains of liability when care or coverage go awry for some reason, and the more insistently will alliances, plans, and networks build their legal staffs and cover their flanks in a kind of preventive and defensive legal medicine. Quasi-public entities such as alliances often occupy a legal twilight zone and, even as explicated by federal laws and rules, will require assimilation into the traditions and codes of the fifty states. Don Kettl captured the problem vividly (if inelegantly): "These liability issues are like a clogged sewer pipe: the question is into whose basement will it back up?"

HEALTH PLANS. To do their jobs well, alliances will need access to abundant data that capture the main dimensions of plan performance. Presumably they will get these data from the health plans themselves. But suppose that plans view the reporting requirements as unreasonable and onerous or are unwilling to release proprietary information? And what happens if plans disagree with alliances over the use and interpretation of these data? Data can do little to empower consumers unless they are cleaned, standardized, interpreted, and translated into plain language. There is little reason to assume that the data will speak for themselves or that the plans will decline to do so—loudly—if they conclude that new government bureaucracies are hindering their progress in the marketplace. Nor will the scope of such conflicts be easily confined to plan-government encounters. A vexing question now confronting states moving toward managed competition is how far nonprofit alliances should be subject to sunshine laws requiring information disclosures, public meetings, and open records. If they are managing health insurance purchasing for large segments of the American public, it will be hard to circumscribe the public's right to know all about their business, and, by extension, the business of those with whom they do business.

Alliances, moreover, are expected to hold down costs. They must decline bids that stand more than 20 percent above the regional average and might try to negotiate bidders toward lower rates in order to avoid premium caps and deliver good budgetary news to their boards. This image of negotiating from strength is appealing in theory, but in practice it pits new organizations of uncertain staff depth and capacity against the owners of health plans that may have weathered a pitiless natural selection and survival of the fittest as small, marginal operators fail or consolidate with big, powerful integrated systems. Might not this be a recipe for regulatory capture, especially if (as is entirely possible) the premium caps are thrown overboard in congressional bargaining?

GOVERNMENT. States that are accustomed to paying and arranging for the coverage of their own employees and public clients such as those on medicaid may be reluctant to start buying care for these groups through newly minted nonprofit corporations with ambiguous accountability to the public sector and therewith to the taxpayer. If the alliances do not work well, what is the alternative? (Raising taxes to cover the "fair" share of the cost of the state clients in the pool as determined by the dynamic interplay of alliance and plans is not a comforting answer.) Furthermore, multiple alliances within states could mean significant variations in costs (and perhaps quality and access) among groups of state workers and clients. Interventions to protect the state's special groups may strike resentful alliances and plans as market interference and may look like favoritism to other groups in the pool who are represented by less formidable sponsors. States may think twice before handing a blank check to a black box.

COMMUNITIES. Health alliances would represent a sizable subset of the community in its health insurance purchasing role, but can purchasing be divorced from planning (a task no one seems to want the alliances to perform) in a rapidly changing market? The prospect that the central government might legislate a national strategy for managed competition has ignited a frenzy of institutional repositioning as hospitals, physicians, and insurers seek to stabilize and enlarge their market shares before the brave new world of more exclusive, integrated, and competing networks arrives. Integrated service networks have come into flamboyant fashion, and mergers and acquisitions are triggering new alliances among providers (and between them and insurers) in hopes of bidding for the business—or countervailing the power—of the anticipated health alliances. As consolidation proceeds, might not some communities lose ownership of their facilities and thus perhaps influence over services? If small and medium-sized communities find themselves served by remotely headquartered health plans, and community-based institutional boards cede power to distant power centers, health ceases to be a community affair. Alliances are charged with empowering consumers to exercise market choices, but what if, in the larger scheme of things, that means disempowering communities? Is this a problem about which alliances should worry? If it troubles their boards or constituents, ought they to intercede? If so, how? Can they be expected to stick to pooled purchasing without getting drawn into conflicts over the shape and structure of what is purchased?

Emerging State Alliances: Constrained and Cautious

Academicians and policymakers have vigorously debated for years the merits of managed competition, including versions that prominently feature health alliance-like structures as purchasing agents. Until the 1990s, however, no state had tried to fashion a formal facsimile of this approach, although any was presumably free to do so. Since the fall of 1992, when Bill Clinton declared that managed competition and health insurance purchasing cooperatives were the foundations of his health care reform program, this strategy has been touted as the wave of the future and state-level discussion of it has increased exponentially. It is therefore useful to glance at three states—California, Florida, and Washington—often said to be farthest down the road toward implementing workable health alliances.

California has been the laboratory of democracy's most enthusiastic host for competitive, market-based health care reform proposals, a distinction probably explained by its tradition of multiple, fragmented, competing insurers and the presence for decades of Kaiser-Permanente and other health maintenance organizations (HMOs) and HMO variants. Although the state has not created a formal system of statewide health alliances, some analysts believe that it is well positioned to do so. A consultant to the California Senate Appropriations Committee observed that California has "a large number of organized providers of health care that are out in the population that are competing for enrollees right now." Moreover, employers are accustomed to offering workers a choice of health plans, and employees are familiar with the notion of choice among plans and know which doctors and hospitals are affiliated with which plan.[16]

California also has the California Public Employees' Retirement System (CALPERS), often held up as a prime specimen of a health alliance prototype. CALPERS covers a wide range of state employees and retirees as well as many local public workers, and it bargains with health plans over the cost and terms of coverage. In the last year the system has won national notice and the deep affection of procompetition theorists by holding average rate increases for its enrollees to 1.4 percent. What some attribute to hard-nosed bargaining, however, others credit mainly to state policy itself, which in 1992 capped state contributions to workers' health benefits. CALPERS responded by creating a uniform benefit package with certain required copayments, which in combination with fixed state contributions left workers facing new out-of-pocket costs, thereby creating a new cost consciousness that presumably registered strongly with the board and staff of CALPERS. It is difficult to disentangle the effects of pooled purchasing from those of fiscal incentives built into broader coverage policies and rulings.[17]

After engineering a thoroughgoing reorganization of its health policy agencies, Florida began installing managed competition in 1993 by establishing eleven regional community health purchasing alliances (CHPAs), nonprofit bodies that bargain on behalf of small businesses, state employees, individuals, and medicaid clients.[18] Key political leaders and private stakeholders endorsed the strategy, but insurers, providers, business groups, and many important legislators recoiled from alliances with the power to reshape the system. The small businesses that can join the alliances are those with fifty or fewer workers, and a debate continues over whether those who enroll in them must buy their health insurance through them. Moreover, the alliances are purely voluntary, raising concerns about adverse selection. Policy leaders in Florida view the CHPAs as the last best hope for voluntarism; beyond them supposedly lies an employer mandate. Proponents of the CHPAs hope that they will exert sufficient leverage in the small-group market to drive prices down to a level that entices most small firms to cover their workers. Skeptics doubt that such mechanisms can make a major dent in the problems of a state in which about 23 percent of the population under retirement age lacks coverage and small businesses dominate the economy.

Washington State, like California, is, in some respects, a natural home for health alliances. It is the site of the nation's most prominent and successful cooperative prepaid group practice—the Group Health Cooperative of Puget Sound—and has shown an uncommon taste for health policy leadership in state government. In the 1970s and 1980s, for example, it had the only mandatory program west of the Mississippi for setting hospital rates. In 1993 Washington created four voluntary private health alliances and one public statewide alliance for public employees and clients of public programs. The state plan is a self-insured operation that offers a benchmark against which public and private purchasers can measure the performance (including cost) of private managed-care plans. Whereas Florida appropriated modest subsidies to help launch and run its alliances, Washington's private cooperatives must cover their own costs. How the alliances will fare is anyone's guess. Possible exclusion of plans and providers became a predictably hot political issue, so alliances are obliged to contract with all health plans in their region. Fear of adverse selection against the voluntary alliances remains, and the need for reliable risk-adjustment methods is recognized. And because Washington has also legislated strict community rating, the utility of alliances as bargainers and shoppers in the insurance market remains to be seen.

Conclusion

Health alliances have undeniable appeals, but the more one ponders the challenges of implementing them in fifty states, the less likely it seems that the exercise can be kept simple. A true recipe for frustration would be to implement alliances by a theoretical blueprint captured in detailed national legislation. How alliances look and perform will vary substantially by state and region. A few states may be well prepared for the challenges, but many others have scarcely a clue how to proceed and most fall somewhere in between. A federally mandated choice between health alliances and a single-payer model makes little sense when neither option fits well in two-thirds or more of the states.

We offer three policy suggestions. First, implementation in the states would proceed better if the federal government devised a more coherent sharing of functions: federal policy frameworks should address matters that are truly national, and states should enjoy new flexibility on issues that properly reflect diverse subnational preferences. American federalism today is largely incoherent: the central government shirks tasks it should take on and puts obstacles in the path of states that summon the political will to try to fill the ensuing gaps. For example, equity should be a major federal concern because sizable state-based disparities violate the notion of universal coverage. Federal legislation, therefore, should create a national entitlement to health care, define its content in a basic benefits package, and design a financing system that apportions costs among employers, taxpayers, and households. National uniformity need not entirely exclude state diversity: if Vermont, say, wanted to adopt a single-payer system financed largely by public monies, why not? The federal government should, however, assure that variations do not defeat universality and its implied equity claims.

Efficiency also is a legitimate national objective. Universal coverage should be affordable for both society and individual citizens, which precludes enormous fluctuations in costs and payments across the states. The federal government should therefore establish national mechanisms to help slow the rate of growth of health spending. But states differ in their base costs, market structures, demographics, and policy preferences and ought to be free to experiment, within reasonable limits, with global budgets, managed competition, all-payer rate setting, and variations on these and other themes.

With delivery system issues, the national interest in uniformity grows cloudy. Arguably, the central government should set a general framework of rules to guide state efforts toward such goals as assuring quality and developing medical personnel in underserved areas, but states should be able to decide for themselves how they want to balance generalists, specialists, and nurses, and how much to promote managed care.

This division of labor is more easily sketched than elaborated. True universal coverage means that the whole population—including poor, ill-educated high users of service—has true access to the whole benefit package. Without resorting to micromanagement, can federal bureaucrats write intelligent rules or performance standards that will persuade the states to secure such access? If states are permitted to experiment with diverse cost containment schemes, how many errors (and how large) will be tolerated before the federal government tightens the fiscal screws or demands something new? If a state concludes that developing report cards that supposedly inform consumers about the quality of local health plans is a meaningless exercise, or one for which they are unprepared, should Washington pressure it to see the light? Given that federal-state cooperation can never be detached from partisan and ideological bickering at both levels, can federal agencies be trusted to write performance standards that stop far short of the intrusive mandates that so annoy the states? A better intergovernmental compact is not a moral or technical quest that awaits new infusions of good will among the players or more clever administrative techniques. Federal-state relations are not problems to be solved but rather tensions to be managed. We are not sanguine about the prospect for improvement, but we believe nonetheless that some good might come of more persistent exploration of these issues.

Second, alliances entail adventures in regionalism and federalism that will be difficult to design, implement, and steer unless the states are somehow formally incorporated into governance early on. The newly coherent markets the Clinton plan envisions demand a newly coherent division of labor between the central and state governments; this means something quite different from rigid blueprints and regulations handed down by Washington from on high. The states should be included in creative institutional machinery for bargaining over the shape of a system that will necessarily evolve by trial and error. A national health board, for instance, might explicitly reserve a number of seats for representatives of the states. To be sure, such collective representation is easier said than done, for the fifty states display distinct cultural traditions, partisan preferences, and policy tastes. But timely inclusion of state voices and more prospective attention to implementation issues rest on the same rationale: both make for better policy formulation.

Third, if many states are to pursue the alliance strategy or some facsimile of it, the sooner policymakers dispel illusions of automaticity in implementation, the better. The structural issues surrounding alliances are complex and intensely political. Organizational technologies and capacities may fall short of what is needed. Relations with purchasers, groups, and communities may be rocky. No invisible hand, economic or administrative, will guide them to a happy end. Building successful alliances will require time, money, technical assistance, staff and board development, and, not least important, political commitment by state policymakers.

The nation's track record to date, compiled in such organization-building endeavors as health maintenance organizations, professional standards review organizations, and health systems agencies, offers little ground for optimism. These institutions were generally adopted as regional and local lowest common denominators on which diverse parties and ideologies could compromise. They were then allowed to proceed out of sight and out of mind with little nourishment until negative evaluations triggered modifications or abandonment. There is little political payoff for funding and nurturing new quasi-public agencies. Although alliances are the heart of a policy proposal that promises to reorganize the health care system without undue reliance on government, alliances and their complementary institutions will not work well unless government—especially state government—expands and refines its capacities. Establishing and monitoring alliances and their relations with health plans demands significantly upgraded state managerial capacities: more and better-trained staff in health and insurance departments; more and better data and management information systems to process them; and more sophisticated and sustained dialogues among state health officials, alliance boards and staffs, and managers of health plans. But few political leaders care to identify themselves, and the cause of health care reform, with appeals to the electorate to fund more bureaucrats in the state capital to regulate the system. Underinvestment in state management and implementation capacities is penny-wise, pound-foolish, perverse, and predictable.

The problem goes deeper: alliances promise insulation that shields political leaders from the heat of conflict over cost containment and supposedly relieves fears of big government among purchasers, providers, insurers, and the public. Policymakers therefore have sound pragmatic reasons not to become too committed to or identified with the work of the alliances. The political incentives driving the formulation of alliances may stand at odds with the managerial incentives that would help to implement them effectively. Federal flexibility and a clearer state voice in designing the national system may help, but trade-offs between insulation and implementation will persist and will demand abundant sensitivity and engagement from public managers who may get few thanks for their efforts.

3 || Cost Containment and Rate Setting

James W. Fossett

EXPLICIT government action to limit spending has been among the most controversial issues in the debate over health care reform. Proposals to institute formal government controls over health care prices, expenditures, or the cost of insurance have generated strong opposition from provider groups and health industries fearful of losing income and revenue, people fearful of "rationing" and losing access to care, particularly through advanced technology, and business groups distrustful of government and excessive bureaucracy.

As a result of this controversy, enacted or proposed health care reforms differ more on the extent of overt cost containment than on most other matters. Nationally, the Clinton administration proposal, the single-payer bill proposed by Representative Jim McDermott and Senator Paul Wellstone, and Representative Fortney "Pete" Stark's emerging proposal, for example, contain goals for expenditure growth and cost containment provisions of greater or lesser severity, frequently described as backstops to cost reduction through managed competition or other unspecified market forces.[1] Other prominent plans have no explicit growth targets or formal cost control structure. Some proponents of these plans claim that expenditure growth will diminish through the creation of "smarter" markets in which customers are more attuned to differences in quality and cost between providers because they have access to more and better information and bear a greater share of the cost of insurance.

States' experiences with explicit cost containment efforts have been limited and extremely uneven. Some experimented with hospital rate regulation during the late 1970s, but only a few—most visibly, New York, Massachusetts, New Jersey, and Maryland—have continued regulation at varying scales. More recently some state health care reforms have incorporated cost containment features that resemble those of the administration plan—reliance on managed competition with more coercive measures if market changes are ineffective. Even in these states overt cost containment has been controversial and has been achieved, as one contributor to this volume has argued elsewhere, through the presence of liberal groups of sufficient strength to make viable threats of more radical changes if modest changes were resisted.[2] In most states the political and judicial legitimacy of large-scale overt regulation of health expenditures has yet to be established.

These observations suggest that the successful institutionalization of cost containment will be among the most difficult political and administrative tasks for any national plan. Cost containment will prove politically difficult to sustain because it takes money out of providers' pockets and may result in the closure of facilities that are major employers and purchasers in local areas. Creating institutions that can reduce growth in health care spending against considerable political opposition from those who see their jobs and incomes at risk is a type of task with which the American system has little successful experience.

Cost containment will also prove difficult administratively because it involves tasks at which Americans have little collective practice. Politicians, providers, and payers have little experience with the bargaining and other political interactions that international experience suggests is necessary for successful implementation of such a plan. The judicial legitimacy of this means of regulation remains to be established, and the information infrastructure necessary to support informed regulation of either expenditures or revenues is largely absent.

This chapter examines the issues likely to arise in the implementation and administration of health cost containment on a large scale. Given the frequent political representation of cost containment as a backstop or club to be used if market forces fail to produce an acceptable decline in the rate of growth in health spending, I first examine the likelihood that market forces—defined here as a rapid diffusion of managed care with or without managed competition in various forms—are likely to achieve major reductions in health care spending in the short time frames contemplated in most proposals. I then examine two generic cost containment methods—expenditure regulation, as practiced in many European countries and partially in several American contexts, and revenue regulation, as contemplated in the Clinton administration's proposal and recently implemented in several states.

The Possibilities for Managed Care or Competition

The widespread opposition to formal cost containment proposals has led many advocates to describe them as backstops or insurance that may not be needed at all or will be instituted if market forces—usually envisioned as managed care or, in the Clinton plan, managed competition—are ineffective in reducing spending growth below some set of target amounts. For plans such as the administration's that involve a considerable expansion of federal government spending to support the purchase of insurance or other subsidies, these targets must be extremely rigorous in order to make the proposal budget neutral under the PAYGO rules attached to the congressional budget process, which require that any additional entitlement spending be offset by savings or additional revenue.[3] The Stark plan has less ambitious targets and provides an as yet unspecified grace period before price controls are instituted.[4]

This need to meet the PAYGO targets and the political need to minimize the invasiveness of expenditure controls requires that administration spokespersons, or advocates of any other plan requiring considerable additional spending, make extremely strong claims about the ability of managed care or competition to get large savings out of the system in a very short time.[5] Recent analyses of the growth targets in the Clinton proposal, for example, have estimated that they would reduce the rate of real per capita growth in health costs from 4 to 5 percent a year to 1.5 percent by 1996 and essentially to zero by 2000.[6] This is a very sharp reduction in a very short time to a growth rate that is much below the average of even heavily regulated health care systems in other industrialized countries in the past thirty years.[7]

It seems improbable that such a dramatic reduction can be achieved so quickly either through broader use of managed care, the most widely practiced method of cost containment, or through managed competition, which attempts to introduce greater market incentives into health care decisions. Experience provides little cause for confidence that managed-care organizations would make such a strong impact so quickly.

First, many states will be virtually starting from scratch in developing such organizations. Enrollment growth in managed care has increased from 60 percent of insured employees in 1987 to 95 percent in 1990.[8] The overwhelming share of growth, however, has come in managed fee-for-service plans in which providers accept discounted fees in exchange for a guaranteed flow of patients. Enrollment in health maintenance organizations, particularly group and staff-model HMOs, which have shown the most consistent success in providing lower cost care, has remained virtually flat and geographically localized on the two coasts and in several states in the Midwest.[9] Even in these states, HMO enrollment does not exceed one-third of the insured population.[10] In other states, particularly in the South and lower Midwest, HMOs remain a curiosity. Large employers, which have been among the most aggressive advocates of managed care, are relatively rare in these states, hostility among providers to nontraditional practice forms remains high, and medical and other provider societies are among the most powerful interest groups.[11] In these states putting the necessary organizations in place is likely to be an extended and difficult process. Private managed-care companies are more likely to be able to respond more quickly than government agencies would be.

Second, the record of managed care in sharply reducing the growth rate of health expenditures is not encouraging. Group or staff-model HMOs, the most invasive and least popular form of managed care, can provide care 10 to 15 percent more cheaply than a fee-for-service system, but much of the savings appears to result from one-time reductions in hospital use rather than a permanent reduction in growth rates. Less regulated but more popular forms of managed care, such as regulated fee for service, have been less effective in achieving even one-time savings.[12]

Advocates of managed competition argue that the limited effectiveness of managed care in reducing cost growth could be improved by altering the tax treatment of health insurance so that households see more of the cost of additional insurance above some minimal package and are required to pay for it with after-tax dollars.[13] And, they contend, by encouraging competition between health plans through the alliance system and providing consumers with more information about the cost and quality of competing plans, managed competition can provide strong incentives for providers and customers to pay more attention to cost. These changes might result in appreciable savings, as some consumers decide not to purchase unsubsidized coverage and plans develop innovative, more cost-effective means of providing care in order to increase market share. Administration spokespersons, for example, argue that aggressive efforts by some states and large corporations to become more activist and innovative purchasers in ways that go well beyond conventional managed-care arrangements is evidence that greater competition might produce more savings than traditional managed care has been able to achieve.[14]

Although speculation is difficult, even a rapidly implemented system of managed competition is unlikely to achieve nonincremental reductions in spending growth. Individual companies or managed-care organizations may have been able to achieve impressive reductions in spending, but because of self-selection among current patients and providers, these results may not be accurate guides to the savings that can be expected nationally or in any particular area.[15] Patients and providers are very often affiliated with managed-care organizations as a result of choice and may be more willing than patients and providers outside these organizations to accept the associated limitations on practice patterns and income. The group and staff-model HMOs and other organizations that have been the most successful at reducing costs have emphasized recruiting providers who support managed care or whose practice patterns are consistent with an emphasis on cost-effective care.[16] Incorporating patients who do not support managed care or providers who practice in a fashion incompatible with it may make universal managed care less effective in reducing costs than are organizations staffed by providers who have voluntarily selected this mode of practice.

Logistical and political difficulties may also limit the effectiveness of managed competition. Advocates of managed competition and other commentators have argued that competition between plans is likely to be most effective when providers are exclusively affiliated with one plan rather than with several, as is currently the case in many areas. Exclusive affiliation eliminates the possibility of cost shifting from one purchaser to another and may encourage more efficient use of resources.[17]

Exclusive affiliation may be demographically difficult to achieve in some states and politically difficult in others. Many rural and smaller urban areas lack the population to support competing plans. And about 30 percent of the metropolitan area population resides in market areas with populations of less than 180,000, which has been identified as the threshold below which extensive sharing of in-patient facilities between provider groups would be necessary. In only ten states does more than half the population reside in market areas of 1.2 million people, the minimum number estimated to support as many as three fully independent competing plans.[18] Under these conditions, exclusive affiliation is likely to be difficult to achieve and the possibility of considerable cost shifting will still exist.

Even in states where managed care is nominally well established, HMOs and other purchasers are frequently subject to legislative restrictions, enacted at the behest of provider groups, that limit their scope of operation and their ability to regulate provider behavior or discriminate in referrals.[19] Among the more common restrictions are "any willing provider" statutes, which limit the ability of managed-care agencies to steer patients to particular providers, and limits on the use of primary care physicians as gatekeepers to control access to specialists, utilization review, and so-called point-of-service plans. Provider groups in states that have undertaken health care reforms have already begun to seek similar legislative restrictions on the operations of health care plans to limit the plans' ability to restrict access to their enrollees and weaken their bargaining leverage.[20] These statutes and the fear of litigation under antitrust or other statutes may have limited more aggressive cost containment actions by managed-care organizations.

Available evidence thus suggests that market forces probably cannot achieve a quick reduction in the rate of growth in health care costs. The organizational infrastructure to enroll large numbers of people in a short time does not exist in many states, the overall record of managed care in reducing cost growth is uneven, and demographic and political conditions may offset some of the alleged cost advantages of managed competition. Although particular companies, purchasing arrangements, or organized delivery systems may well be able to achieve impressive reductions in cost, others will almost certainly be less successful, making it likely that any backup formal cost containment system will be invoked.

Cost Containment Alternatives

A wide variety of schemes have been proposed and attempted to control health expenditures, but most proposals under serious consideration involve one of two generic approaches. One, practiced in various forms both in this and other industrialized countries and best typified in the current debate by the McDermott-Wellstone single-payer bill, is the direct regulation of expenditures or the amount paid to particular providers. A national board would set a national health budget and divide it among the states, which would be responsible for administering it within their borders. The other type of plan, best exemplified by the Clinton administration's proposal or reform schemes adopted in Washington State and Minnesota, regulates revenues by restricting the amount of money that can be collected in premiums from employers and households, with the method of payment to particular providers left to individual plans.

Particular versions of these two schemes may look more alike than different, and many plans have aspects of both. Recent experiments in expenditure control, for example, have emphasized global budgeting, regulating total spending rather than the rates for individual services or procedures, an approach that resembles a revenue cap. By contrast, the Clinton administration's plan, as well as recent reforms in Washington State and Minnesota, relies primarily on regulating growth in the premiums that can be paid to competing plans, but also prescribes fee schedules, or expenditure regulation, for physicians who remain in fee-for-service practices. These generic approaches differ appreciably, however, in the process by which caps are set and apportioned among individual providers, the politics surrounding this process and, allegedly, in their effectiveness.

Regulating Expenditures

Health expenditures have typically been controlled in this country and elsewhere through regulation of payments to providers, usually through a prospective process that translates a lump sum set by the political process into payments to individual providers. This lump sum can be subdivided into allocations for geographic areas, divided among particular provider sectors such as hospitals or physicians, allocated directly to individual providers through the development of rates or fee schedules for individual procedures or services, or some combination of these procedures.[21]

Expenditure control systems in Europe and Canada have relied on complex combinations of these methods, but generally budgets are negotiated directly with individual hospitals, and physicians' fee schedules are negotiated between provincial health ministries and physicians' organizations.[22] American experience, which has been more limited, has centered on the regulation of rates, largely for inpatient hospital care, through the development of statistical formulas to establish the fees for individual services to be charged to payers.[23] American systems of expenditure regulation at both federal and state levels have historically covered only parts of the health care system, particularly hospitals, or particular groups of patients. They have thus allowed considerable shifting of expenditures to unregulated patients or sites of care.[24] Although American systems are largely still tied to regulating fees rather than total expenditures, there is increasing experimentation in several locations with global budgeting, which regulates total expenditures rather than the prices and quantities of particular services.[25]

Bureaucratic and legislative debates over rate setting are heavily dominated by considerations of providers' financial condition rather than the level of resources available, and demands for accommodation of labor settlements or other localized problems are frequently made and agreed to. As in the case of many other price-setting regulatory systems, most systems also allow appreciable incumbent protection and contain subsidies for particular groups of facilities whose potential closure is politically or clinically unacceptable. Adjustments to the medicare prospective payment formula for rural and teaching hospitals, for example, have been defended less on their own merits than as a means of getting money to the "right" places.[26] State reimbursement schemes have also frequently been altered to accommodate particular areas or groups of facilities or to provide general deficit relief.[27] As a result, politically successful American rate-setting systems have relied on gradual reductions in the permitted rate of expenditure growth over an extended time. Medicare's prospective payment system, for example, involved an appreciable phase-in period, and Maryland's all-payer system took nine years to reduce costs per admission to the national average from 25 percent above the national figure.[28] In similar fashion New York's several hospital reimbursement systems, which have had more complex objectives, have relied on gradual reductions in growth rates.[29]

Advocates of this approach defend both its record in reducing costs and its political realism in bargaining directly with providers whose compliance is critical to the success of any plan. Although the record and the survival of state systems is decidedly mixed, most assessments of all-payer rate setting have found evidence of reduced growth rates as compared to rates in unregulated states.[30] In similar fashion, the major cost containment goals of medicare's prospective payment system appear to have been realized.[31] Experience in regulating expenditures in Germany and Canada, as well as other regulatory experience in this country, also suggests that close provider involvement in both allocation and compliance has potential advantages.[32] Regulated groups become more vested in a solution if they have had some considerable role in shaping it, and provider groups, particularly physicians, might be more compliant with enforcement efforts by their peers than by state agencies. While such self-regulation likely has a cost in terms of the ability to meet any explicit set of expenditure targets, it may also have many political advantages.[33]

Regulating Revenues: Premium Caps

The Clinton administration's proposed plan and some state health care reform efforts embody a second approach to cost containment that regulates the revenues that organized health plans have available to spend. Although states have the option either to establish a single-payer system or to operate the alliance system under the administration's plan, the major means for securing compliance with growth targets is federal regulation of premiums collected by alliances, thus limiting the amount of money available for health care in each alliance area to a predetermined, fixed amount. A baseline average premium would be set for individual alliances by a federal national health board based on a national average adjusted to reflect differences between alliances in health spending, insurance coverage, and spending by academic medical centers.[34] Subsequent growth in the weighted average premium within each alliance would be tied to consumer inflation and population growth, adjusted for differences in demographic characteristics between alliances.

The national health board would compel reductions in premiums in alliances whose growth rates exceeded permissible levels, and alliances could refuse to accept premium bids from plans that were more than 20 percent above the acceptable rate. Alliances would also be responsible for setting schedules for fee-for-service providers outside health plans. Reforms in Minnesota and Washington State that follow this arrangement have set more permissive goals for premium growth and have relied much more heavily, at least rhetorically, on competition to restrict cost growth.[35]

Although there is little experience with this mode of regulation, advocates have argued that controlling premiums has a number of advantages over regulating expenditures.[36] Regulating average premiums that finance packages of services is said to be more flexible than regulating the prices for individual services and to make it more difficult to manipulate the system to benefit particular providers or other local interests. Advocates also contend that this method is better insulated from state political processes, which have been widely considered unduly responsive to provider interests. The default site for regulating revenues is at the federal level, where providers are presumably less powerful than in individual states. Perhaps most important, dealing with providers, which may involve unpleasant decisions about closing facilities and reducing provider incomes in potentially dramatic ways, is governed by health plans and alliances rather than by the political process. Locating these transactions in the nominally private sector would relieve legislators of the necessity of voting to approve cost containment schemes that might damage large employers and purchasers in their districts. Inefficient providers thus have less recourse than under present regulatory systems, where appeals to the political process are easily pressed.[37]

Implementation Prospects

Either of these methods represents a dramatic increase in the scale and scope of government health care regulatory activity. Although the federal government has considerable experience regulating medicare payments to physicians and hospitals, and half the states have at least some experience with setting in-patient hospital rates, the difference in political and administrative complexity between such limited activities and the regulation of total health care expenditures is considerable. Regulation of hospital in-patient rates, for example, requires supervision of a relatively small number of heavily regulated institutions. Global regulation would expand this supervision to out-patient facilities, private physicians, and a large number of other providers with which states have little experience. In similar fashion, although the federal government has appreciable experience in regulating expenditures, at least for medicare patients, it has little experience in the particulars of regulating revenues or insurance pricing.

There is, in brief, a large difference between experience at either the state or federal level and the administrative and political requirements of either generic cost containment approach. Apart from the administrative difficulties associated with putting the appropriate organizational machinery into place, effective implementation or institutionalization of either scheme requires considerable attention to three major classes of recurring political and administrative problems. The cost containment structure needs sufficient insulation from the political process to be able to reduce the rate of growth in health care costs, it needs some means of dealing with adverse judicial decisions, and it needs some means of resolving contentious technical issues of data and measurement.

Political Insulation

There has been a general presumption that regulatory agencies, both local and federal, charged with overseeing cost containment require some insulation from the normal political process. Appreciable reductions in the rate of growth in health care costs will result in the loss of income for physicians and other providers, may lead to the closure of hospitals or other facilities that are major employers and purchasers, and may lead to large layoffs from public and private payrolls. The parties at risk for these losses have considerable influence with elected officials and might be expected to use this influence to neutralize or penalize agencies attached to normal government departments and financed through the normal budget process.

These potential problems have led reform advocates to propose establishing insulated alliances and state agencies. Typically, insulated agencies, such as the Federal Reserve System, operate outside established state or federal departments, are governed by independently appointed commissions or boards whose members are appointed to long, staggered terms, and are usually financed outside the normal budget process through fees or other earmarked revenue that is not legislatively appropriated. These agencies frequently have discretion over when they take particular actions, and the actions generally do not require formal approval of any outside agency or elected official.

Reform advocates have argued that federal and state health agencies and alliances require similar protection against political interference.[38] The Clinton administration's plan and other managed-competition variants attempt to insulate this process further by placing the decisions outside the political process in negotiations between plans and individual providers.

The insulated agencies most frequently mentioned as models for federal and state health agencies or alliances have behaved in ways constrained in some fashion by a desire to preserve their independent status and thus maintain de facto informal accountability and legitimacy. Formal insulation, if used skillfully, confers considerable tactical autonomy, but it does not eliminate the need for agencies to observe politically defined limits on their actions. Three types of agencies have frequently been mentioned as models for health boards and alliances, arranged roughly in descending order of formal insulation.

FEDERAL RESERVE SYSTEM. The Federal Reserve System is the prototypical insulated agency and the analogy most frequently mentioned for federal and state health board or alliance status and operations. It enjoys much more extensive formal autonomy than do the executive departments of the federal government.[39] It exercises wide discretion over the timing and level of changes in discount and interest rates through a relatively secretive process that requires no initiation or approval by outside forces. Members of the Federal Reserve Board, the system's governing body, are appointed by the U.S. president to fourteen-year staggered terms. The system's budget is financed by assessments on member banks and is approved without review at the level requested by both executive and legislative budget processes, thus limiting the ability of the president or Congress to sanction the Federal Reserve through commonly used devices.

This formal insulation does not insulate it either from external influence or the need to take strategic action calculated to preserve its independence. Several respectable political scientists have, in fact, found statistical evidence of Federal Reserve compliance in "political business cycles" calculated to enhance the reelection prospects of presidential and congressional incumbents.[40] John Woolley's sophisticated assessment of the Federal Reserve's relations with the president and Congress indicates a pattern of "fire fighting" in which "cyclical mobilization and demobilization of political forces provoke shifting responses from the Federal Reserve."[41] Presidents and Congress frequently make attempts to influence Federal Reserve policy; Federal Reserve officials may resist or comply, depending on the political and economic circumstances. The Federal Reserve has considerable political resources in addition to its formal independence, particularly its sizable constituencies in the banking and finance industries, but is susceptible to influence by others, particularly the president. Federal Reserve officials are also attentive to congressional opinion and may be compelled to facilitate the decline of interest rates "around the time that Congress has worked up the anger necessary to take action [to restrict the Federal Reserve's independence]."[42]

MILITARY BASE CLOSING AND REALIGNMENT COMMISSION. A second insulated body is the Military Base Closing and Realignment Commission, first established in 1988 and extended for five years in 1990.[43] The commission process emerged as a means of designating bases to be closed or downsized as a result of conflict between congressional Democrats and the Bush administration and concerns that pork barrel politics would make it impossible for Congress to agree on bases to be closed. The process was intended to remove power from both the executive branch and Congress to prevent or initiate a base closing for political gain by generating, from recommendations submitted by the Department of Defense, a list of bases to be closed or downsized that

Congress could approve or disapprove but not amend.[44] The commission can add or remove facilities from the recommendations of the secretary of defense and has done so in several cases. Three rounds of closings were approved by Congress in 1989, 1991, and 1993, and an additional round is scheduled for 1995. The recommendations of the first two rounds have withstood both judicial challenges and attempts to block closings by failing to appropriate money for them. The 1990 reauthorization act further limited the use of the appropriations process by authorizing the secretary to close or realign bases without regard to contrary language in appropriations acts.

While both the Department of Defense and the commission apply several statutory criteria relating to military value, payback periods, and economic impact in generating recommendations, both have also been sensitive to informal, but clearly understood, criteria of fairness between parties, regions of the country, and the various services. Lobbying of individual services, the secretary of defense, and commission members and staff has been increasingly vigorous and has resulted in bases being removed or added. The commission attempted in 1991 to expand its mandate by recommending major changes in the district structure of the Army Corps of Engineers, but this proposal, unlike recommendations on the closing of bases, was blocked in the appropriations process.

The Base Closing Commission provides a useful case of the tactical rather than the strategic value of insulation. Only a limited number of congressional districts are adversely affected in any given round, which minimizes potential opposition to the commission's recommendations. Congressional inability to amend recommendations or block the appropriation of funds to implement closures severely lessens the strength of opposition. This insulation by packaging and procedure, as well as the commission's ability to modify the recommendations of the secretary of defense, provides the commission with considerable tactical freedom, but has not eliminated the necessity to observe the limits on its mandate and informal but widely understood norms of fairness about the distribution of closures.

PUBLIC AUTHORITIES AND RATE-SETTING AGENCIES. Other possible models for state agencies or alliances are public authorities or commissions that exist in many states to regulate industries or provide specialized financing of various kinds. These agencies are frequently accountable to appointed or elected commissions rather than government departments, are sometimes exempt from state civil service regulations, and are frequently financed from earmarked revenues such as assessments on the regulated industry or bond proceeds. Previous state efforts at all-payer rate setting often were organized as independent agencies along these lines rather than being incorporated in health departments or other government agencies.

At the risk of oversimplification, comparison of these agencies and government departments that perform the same functions suggests that there is no simple relationship between formal insulation and actual independence from the political process nor any simple connection between formal status and effectiveness, broadly understood. Authorities governed by such aggressive entrepreneurs as Robert Moses have been independent power centers outside the control of elected officials.[45] Others, which have been financing shells created to evade state constitutional debt limits or voter approval requirements, are under the close control of elected officials and state budget offices.[46] Conversely, the structure for regulating hospital rates in New York has benefited from its location in the state Department of Health, while a similar department-based structure in Massachusetts has been hindered by this structure.[47]

Perhaps more important, there appears to be no simple relationship between organizational structure and effectiveness. Allegations of "capture" by agency constituents are pervasive in discussions of state regulatory agencies, but the factors often associated with capture—low agency salaries, high staff turnover, inadequate resources, excessive dependence on regulated industries for information, and lack of organized opposition to industry requests—have no necessary connection with being part of a government department rather than an independent commission.[48] Of the four all-payer rate agencies that survived the early 1980s, for example, three—in New Jersey, New York, and Massachusetts—are located in state departments, while only one—in Maryland—is a commission.

Conditions at least in some states may have become more politically favorable to effective agency operation. Particularly in those states in the Northeast and the West where all-payer rate systems, certificate of need (CON) systems, and other regulatory structures survived the antiregulatory movement of the early 1980s, provider groups have become increasingly divided and conflicts between employers, insurance companies, and providers have become more visible.[49] Under these conditions the odds of agency capture are sharply diminished, and bureaucratic influence over health care is more likely to be substantial.

In other states, particularly in the South, political conditions are less favorable for successful agency operation. Provider groups are still extremely powerful. In some states, appointments of health commissioners and other top officials are made from nominations by medical societies. Many departments are governed by commissions whose appointments are dominated by provider interests. And there is little significant organized opposition to provider groups. Executive and regulatory institutions are traditionally weak, and government salaries and budgets small. Under these conditions, the odds of agency capture are high, and state agencies or alliances, regardless of their formal status, are likely to experience considerable political difficulties. Progress in reducing health care costs along the lines envisioned in any of the proposals currently on the table is likely to be slow at best.

These considerations also suggest that the value of insulating decisions from the political process by making them nominally market decisions may be more apparent than real. Providers, both collectively and individually, have shown themselves adept at using the political process to influence current market structures and payment systems to their advantage, and it seems unlikely that these efforts would diminish with the institution of alliances.

Judicial Insulation

A second problem that cost containment plans will have to confront is the increasing role of federal courts in health reimbursement issues. Most regulatory schemes have undergone extensive judicial scrutiny of their processes and operations, as well as frequent review of particular decisions, and it seems unlikely that either cost containment approach could avoid extensive judicial review at several levels. Although medicare's hospital payment system is exempt by statute from the jurisdiction of federal courts, for example, courts have accepted for judicial determination a wide variety of technical rate-setting matters in state systems and medicaid programs. Most past and existing regulatory schemes have been heavily litigated and frequently appreciably altered by court decisions. The New Jersey rate-setting system was largely invalidated by a federal district court on the grounds that it was preempted by the

Employee Retirement Income Security Act (ERISA), and a major portion of the New York system was recently eliminated on similar grounds.[50] State efforts at cost containment in the medicaid program have likewise been subject to frequent judicial challenges, most commonly on grounds of conflicts with the Boren amendment, which requires hospitals and nursing homes to be paid "reasonable and adequate" medicaid rates.[51] Courts have compelled states to increase medicaid fees to comply with statutory mandates to ensure medicaid pediatric and obstetric patients access to care on a level with the population as a whole.[52] They have also invalidated state attempts to institute copayments and other means of reducing medicaid costs.

Judicial micromanagement of the particulars of budgeting schemes presents a potentially severe obstacle to effective containment of health costs. Since litigation, like war, is the pursuit of politics by other means, both providers and client groups might be expected to challenge cost containment schemes judicially on whatever grounds appear available and convenient to recover in the courts what they lose in the regulatory process. ERISA and the Boren amendment are currently popular grounds for challenging reimbursement schemes, but appropriate legislative corrections, which are proposed in the administration's plan, may only shift the grounds on which suits are brought. Courts have repeatedly overruled, for example, attempts by health maintenance organizations and other insurers to limit payment for experimental or other treatments deemed medically unnecessary and frequently assessed large damages for bad faith against insurers.[53] Such awards should be expected to continue, as should suits under the Americans with Disabilities Act and other legislation that provides preferential access to care for some defined group.

Judicial challenges to the cost containment apparatus on procedural and other grounds developed in other areas of regulation are also likely. The decisions of most regulatory agencies are governed by elaborate sets of procedural rules, growing in large measure out of the Administrative Procedures Act, so that they make decisions that can be defended as reasonable in procedurally appropriate ways. These requirements have been widely argued to unduly complicate and prolong regulatory processes and discourage reliance on politically and administratively effective market processes, bargaining, and other decentralized and informal cooperative processes upon which many current and proposed schemes rely heavily.[54]

Although it is difficult to predict the extent to which judges will insist on applying the same set of requirements to the health cost containment apparatus as to other rate-setting bodies, it seems likely that health plans and providers will press claims on these grounds. The administration's bill, for example, exempts the rate-setting actions of the proposed health board from judicial or administrative review but allows for judicial review of sanctions imposed on alliances or plans and does not appear to exempt the actions of alliances in negotiating with plans or in rejecting premium bids from plans that are unacceptably high. Suits can be expected from rejected plans claiming that alliances are in fact governmental bodies that should be subject to this set of procedures and alleging that rejection of their bid constitutes a violation of Fifth Amendment rights without a fair hearing.[55] If courts are receptive to these claims, the effectiveness of the regulatory structure would be severely compromised.

In addition to these direct effects the possibility of litigation may also hamper the flexible, informal, negotiated local arrangements contemplated under the cost containment systems. European systems that involve extensive provider participation are subject to only the most limited judicial review, meaning that decisions are generally final and the incentives to bargain are strong. When the possibility of litigation and judicial assignment of liability is high or uncertain, however, parties may be less willing to bargain or cooperate informally for fear of compromising their eventual legal position.[56] Such concerns have been identified as important obstacles to successful informal cooperation in other areas, such as the use of "alternative dispute resolution" techniques to mediate environmental disputes.[57] Because there is likely to be an extended period of legal uncertainty while the rights and privileges of various parties are established judicially, it may be inordinately difficult to establish the informal, noncontractual relations common in European systems.

Measurement

A third problem in implementing the regulation of either revenues or expenditures is the difficulty of measuring the level and distribution of health expenditures and calculating legally or politically reasonable measures of whatever differences between providers or patients are recognized by the regulatory scheme. Experience in both Europe and this country indicates that regulation, whether of revenues or expenditures, is an extremely data-intensive enterprise. Agencies that regulate expenditures must be able to measure health care spending inside their borders, compare it to annual targets on a timely basis, and monitor spending for whatever substate entities are assigned targets or caps. Physician reimbursement schemes such as medicare's resource-based relative value system (RBRVS) that adjusts fees in response to changes in volume or complexity require larger volumes of more sophisticated information with very short turnaround times. Physician reimbursement schemes in Germany and some Canadian provinces, for example, that distribute payments quarterly rely heavily on elaborate profiles for individual physicians that report on billing, case mix, services, and a variety of other matters.[58] Medicare's rate systems also require adjustments of basic payment amounts for geographic differences in hospital and medical practice costs and a variety of other factors, and the operation of the program's volume performance standards requires complex calculations of how physicians have adjusted workload volumes in response to fees.

The data and measurement requirements for revenue regulation differ slightly but are equally complex. Setting an adequate base year premium for individual alliances requires that the revenue generated from the premium be roughly equivalent to expenditures, which requires that expenditures be known with a fair degree of confidence. Methods for adjusting benchmark premiums and computing inflation updates for alliances, which will require extensive data for substate areas on health expenditures, insurance status, demographic characteristics, and health status, must also be specified. In addition, the national health board will have to specify methods for risk-adjusting premium payments to individual plans and setting premiums for households that have been previously uninsured.

The ability to meet even the most modest of these goals is almost completely absent in current expenditure-reporting systems. National expenditures can be estimated with a fair degree of precision, and the Health Care Financing Administration has recently published the first annual estimates of state personal health expenditures since 1985.[59] It is uncertain, however, whether these estimates are solid enough to serve as a basis for a budgetary allocation. The ability to measure or monitor expenditures in individual states currently ranges from limited to nonexistent. The few states that operate hospital rate-setting systems collect detailed data on in-patient expenditures and have reasonable estimates about the magnitude of spending for outpatient services, but have only the most perfunctory information on spending in physicians' offices, free-standing care centers, medical equipment vendors, or other locations. Most states lack even this limited information. An increasing number maintain hospital discharge databases, but these systems range in quality from good to awful.

In recognition of these problems, reform efforts in states such as Minnesota and Washington have included considerable investment in developing and collecting a wide range of data to be used in expenditure tracking and cost containment. In similar fashion the administration's bill contains a provision for the development of a comprehensive national health information data system within two years. This time frame appears unreasonably short because assembling information into coherent and comparable information systems that agencies can use to set premiums or track expenditures or both appears to be one of the more tedious and demanding logistical tasks associated with health care reform. Data on expenditures by public programs such as medicare and medicaid exist in theory, but not in anything approaching comparable or usable form. Medicare data appear to have improved appreciably in the last several years, but medicaid data in most states are of extremely poor quality.[60] State medicaid agencies report spending in a number of service categories to receive federal reimbursement, and they submit reports on expenditures and service usage for various separate client groups, but the systems that produce these reports are inconsistent within states in the same year, across states, and over time.[61] Arranging data from medicaid financial reporting systems into forms that are usable for other purposes is expensive, time-consuming, and tedious, and only a few states have invested any appreciable effort along these lines.[62]

The largest obstacle to developing adequate reporting systems is, of course, the large number of private insurance companies that currently make payments to providers on the basis of billings that are of unknown, but likely variable, quality and almost certainly are not comparable in any particular. European systems that make payments through single payers can readily capture all billings by a given provider and make efforts to improve the quality of submissions. But the large number of payers in this country, the limited agreement on data standards, and pervasive incompatibilities between forms, software, and other system particulars suggest that developing the ability to measure expenditures and use is likely to be an expensive, difficult, and lengthy task.[63]

Some idea of the potential time frame of such an enterprise in a large state comes from the Single Payer Demonstration in New York, which required a year to get 28 hospitals connected to an "electronic clearing-house" of the type required to track expenditures with a reasonable degree of sophistication. In interviews, state officials have estimated that connecting all 300-plus hospitals in the state to this system will take five years and considerably longer to establish similar links with the state's more than 50,000 physicians. To cite another recent example, Minnesota took several years to get what it estimates are two-thirds of expenditures, and it plans an extensive multiyear effort to collect all data required.[64]

There is also considerable technical uncertainty and controversy about the most appropriate way to adjust payments and premiums to recognize differences between various providers or patients. The most visible of these measurement issues in the discussion of the Clinton plan, for example, has been the problem of how to risk-adjust premium payments to individual plans to avoid the segregation of poor or sick patients into a small number of plans. A number of observers have argued that existing methods for making these adjustments are inadequate to reflect differences in usage among high- and low-risk groups.[65] Similar technical concerns have been raised about methods for setting premiums for people currently uninsured.[66]

These problems of data and measurement technology are likely to become recurrent political and judicial issues, complicating the process of setting budgets and stretching out compliance with budget or premium growth targets. The administration's plan, for example, attempts to regulate noninvasively and leave as much scope as possible to local negotiations and competition. The problematic nature of the baseline, the difficulty of gauging the appropriateness of adjustments to the growth target, and the possibility that plans will fail to comply with targets because of adverse selection resulting from inadequate risk adjustment rather than inefficiency, however, all suggest that premium setting is likely to be lengthier and more contentious than envisioned. Similar data and measurement questions have become recurrent points of political or judicial contention in other regulatory areas, and it seems unrealistic to expect that they will be avoided in the regulation of health expenditures.[67] The implementation of medicare's volume performance standards, for example, has been marked by sharp conflict over predictions about how physicians will respond to fee changes.[68] States, alliances, and plans will have strong incentives to push for liberal adjustments to both base and growth rates and to blame plan failures on inadequate adjustments for growth and risk.

A second set of data and measurement issues relates to the ability to monitor use and access, particularly by lower-income and high-risk groups. The interest of public agencies in cost containment is balanced by concerns that reduced cost growth will result from improvements in service delivery and the elimination of unnecessary care rather than from risk selection and underserving expensive, hard-to-reach populations. The administrative and technical problems associated with risk-adjusting premiums, which in theory eliminates the incentive for providers to choose the most healthy clients, indicates that even the most market-oriented structures are likely to need considerable detailed reporting on use and access by particular population groups.

This monitoring is likely to prove administratively and politically easier under expenditure regulation systems, where payment is more closely linked to the provision of service and the regulatory structure deals more directly with hospitals and other providers, than it will be under revenue regulation, where payment is based on enrollment rather than usage and contact is filtered through a plan's administrative management. Experience in medicaid managed-care plans and in such states as Minnesota that have chosen systems that resemble the administration's suggests that these requirements are more difficult to negotiate and implement. Plan managers may not use the same measures for the same population groups in their internal control processes, and concerns about the validity of reports may compel regulators to pursue more consensual strategies in the development of reporting requirements, which may lengthen the time required to put these systems into place.

How Fast Can Costs Be Managed Down?

This combination of difficult and cumbersome technical and administrative problems, judicial micromanagement, and potential political problems suggests that federal national health boards are likely to find aggressive enforcement of growth rates and the imposition of penalties for noncompliance politically difficult. Although these agencies can be vested with significant enforcement powers in statute, experience suggests these penalties will be used gingerly, if at all. The Clinton administration's proposed health board, for example, is vested with the ability to reduce payments to noncomplying plans or alliances and reduce payments for medical education and other purposes to recalcitrant states, as well as the power to operate the alliance system in nonparticipating states and levy a 15 percent tax for administrative costs. The very real technical difficulties associated with putting these plans in place, the very real possibility that sanctions may do more harm than good, as well as the desire to avoid either being blamed for shutting down hospitals or taking over alliances, all suggest that what is legislated as an expenditure cap may be enforced as a target under which states or alliances that are "making progress" are unlikely to be penalized. The wide variety among states in the capacity to put data and other systems in place, the political support for cost containment as compared to other goals, the power of providers, and the controversy likely to surround the institution of cost containment policies all suggest that progress toward cost reduction is likely to be slow and uneven regardless of what method is chosen.

These same factors also argue for aggressive federal enforcement. State political systems have difficulty in executing cost containment policies. All-payer rate regulation did not survive in most states that tried it, and those systems that have survived have had to accept considerable incumbent protection as the political price for slow and incremental reductions in the rate of cost growth. In similar fashion, recent state health care reforms have underemphasized cost containment compared to other goals for reasons that are largely political. Provider groups are more powerful in the states than in Washington and have shown themselves willing to deal meaningfully with state decisionmakers only to the extent that they perceive the alternatives as worse. Federal willingness to use sanctions, at least against the most recalcitrant states, is likely to be a critical ingredient in the success of cost containment.

A third problem is the difficulty of sticking to simple decision rules. Many of the expenditure and revenue regulation schemes on the table follow prevailing regulatory wisdom and try to regulate as few things as possible—total expenditures and the package of services the expenditures are to finance. Translating these totals into payments to particular providers for services to particular patients is left to be worked out through local bargaining and negotiation, either in a market context or through more overtly political mechanisms. This posture of regulating only the aggregates and leaving as much as possible to be determined by the affected parties locally has considerable appeal in health care, where, as one observer has contended, "all politics is local politics, but health care politics is *really* local politics."[69]

Much of American regulatory history suggests this simplicity is difficult to maintain because of the political, judicial, and technical need to make exceptions. The decentralized bargaining that both cost containment schemes attempt to encourage is an acceptable means of allocating resources if, as one prominent student of regulation has argued, "agreement itself and not its precise substantive details is of particular importance."[70] Pressures from local losers through state and federal political processes, the possibility of adverse judicial decisions and the need to make procedurally and substantively reasonable judgments that are defensible in court, the technical and data uncertainties associated with important measurements, and concerns about adequate access, quality, and risk selection will all create considerable incentives for whatever cost containment structure is put in place to concern itself with "precise substantive details" in particular areas. Avoiding the tendency toward procedural and technical complexity that has plagued other regulatory arenas will be extremely difficult.

The political advantages of insulation, whether through most favored agency status or through the market process, are more tactical than strategic. Insulation offers short-run packaging and procedural advantages, but both the Federal Reserve System and the Base Closing Commission follow election returns and engage in coalition building and activity calculated to maintain their independence and legitimacy. It is to be expected that both state and federal agencies would engage in similar behavior even if they were to be insulated from attacks on their budget or other overt political threats. Currently, for example, rate-setting systems contain provisions for procedural appeals, holding facilities harmless, and modifications for changes in volume, case mix, and other factors to permit targeted adjustments for particular facilities. The justification for such adjustments is partly technical, but they also provide a means for agency officials to be responsive to what they see as legitimate local concerns. Even under the market-driven system contemplated by the Clinton plan and other managed-competition proposals, alliances and the structure for setting premiums may well find it politically sensible to be responsive as a means of protecting their continued existence.

There is also the potential for continued conflict between the political and financial requirements of the health care reform process and those of the budget process. Politically and administratively successful cost containment is likely to require a long time to put the organizational framework of reform into place and initiate efforts at developing appropriate data and measurement systems. This initial period may be followed by slow and uneven but perhaps increasingly steady incremental reductions in the rate of cost growth. This pattern conflicts with the budget process, which requires that additional expenditures be financed with a greater degree of certainty over a shorter time.

There is no clear basis for judging either generic cost containment plan more readily implementable, at least in the short to medium run. There is more collective experience with expenditure regulation schemes in this country and elsewhere, and the administrative, technical, and political issues likely to arise under such a system are better known and can be more readily addressed. There is less experience with revenue regulation, and more difficulty in generalizing credibly from the experience of a limited number of highly visible managed-care organizations, companies, and purchasing organizations. The very limited amount of experience with such tasks as monitoring risk selection, developing means of risk adjustment, and the other management tasks associated with managed competition suggests that the start-up period is likely to be appreciably longer for a system that regulates revenues rather than expenditures.

Conclusions about the relative effectiveness of these two approaches in reducing the rate of growth in health care costs are more difficult to draw. Decisionmakers are contemplating choices not merely between these alternatives, but between versions of the two alternatives that may differ widely in their effectiveness. A nominal revenue regulation system, for example, under which health plans lack the ability to discriminate among providers and attempts to risk-adjust premiums are seen as technical and political failures, may prove to be more heavily regulated than many expenditure regulation systems, where the governmental role is nominally larger. Public managers under both types of plans will confront strong political, judicial, and technical incentives to micromanage and will have to cope with political and legal challenges from losers and other groups intent on manipulating the system to secure financial or other advantages. Decisionmakers contemplating this choice should focus at least as much on the extent to which the particular proposals in front of them address these problems as on the ideological virtues of the schemes.

This focus on common implementation problems should not, however, obscure the real differences between these two approaches.[71] Managed competition and revenue regulation rely more heavily, at least initially, on "private" rules for assigning patients and allocating care and on holding plans accountable largely on the basis of whether customers are willing to continue to remain enrolled. Under these rules, potential problems with access, risk selection, and the distribution of the burden of cost containment are appreciably more difficult to monitor and address. Expenditure regulation systems, by contrast, rely more heavily on "public" rules set more visibly through the political process. Distributive concerns about access and burdens are more readily addressed under such rules but at the potential price of creating entitlements to continued existence for providers and weakened incentives for innovations and improvements in the efficiency of services. Choices about cost containment may ultimately be driven by the type of mistake one is willing to tolerate.

4 ‖ The Quest for Quality Care: Implementation Issues

Frank J. Thompson

AT LEAST three core values compete for attention in the politics of health care reform: access to care, cost containment, and quality. A nagging suspicion persists that if any two of these are obtained under comprehensive reform it will be difficult to achieve the third. Since the major proposals, including President Clinton's, promise greater access and cost containment, the question remains: will quality get lost in the shuffle?

Some experts say no. Two general reasons undergird this conviction. First, comprehensive health plans would greatly reduce the number of citizens with substandard or no insurance. Because providers would receive comparable compensation for treating all classes of people, they would have less incentive to sacrifice quality for patients who could not pay their bills. Second, comprehensive reform typically promises to exorcise from the health care system costs that do not contribute to quality and may even erode it. Vast amounts of paperwork would presumably vanish from day-to-day medical operations, thus paring administrative overhead. Incentives could be structured to discourage physicians from providing too much care, a practice that not only wastes money but can be dangerous. For instance, people who enter hospitals run some risk that the encounter will lead them to develop new diseases.

Although considerable evidence supports these assertions, hard challenges await those seeking to assure quality in a universal health care

This chapter benefited greatly from the insights of the other authors in this volume and state officials who attended the Rockefeller Institute conference and subsequent meetings at the Brookings Institution. I am especially indebted to Joe White, Beryl Radin, Margaret Stanley, Ray Sweeney, and David Maxwell-Jolly for their comments on an earlier version.

system. Meeting these challenges depends in part on acquiring greater technical sophistication, such as a better understanding of the outcomes of different health care interventions. But the quest for quality assurance is also about federalism, the design and capacity of public and private institutions, and implementation. It is about a politics, substantially centered in vast and dispersed administrative agencies, that plays out after a comprehensive reform bill becomes law. These issues of bureaucratic politics and management will profoundly shape who gets care of what quality in a reformed health care system.[1]

This chapter uses President Clinton's proposed Health Security Act as a springboard to analyze one approach to quality assurance in a universal health care system. Specifically, I analyze three general tenets of the Clinton plan: that assuring quality requires action to make health care markets substantially more informed through, among other things, report cards for plans and providers; that sustaining quality requires enhanced promulgation of practice guidelines grounded in outcomes research; and that fostering quality requires active efforts to open up channels for consumers to voice their views.

Certain basic questions guide my assessment of each of these principles of the Clinton plan. Could the provisions be implemented in a timely and effective manner? Would they have the desired effects? Would an alternative approach to the task make more sense? Does each initiative strike the right balance in terms of the intergovernmental division of labor?

Obviously, the dance of legislation in Washington may ultimately produce a law vastly different from Clinton's proposal, and it may even produce no legislation at all. In either case, however, there is still some benefit from examining the Clinton proposal. In one form or another, the basic issues the bill presents about more informed markets, outcomes research and practice guidelines, and mechanisms for expressing consumer voice will be a part of the policy debate in the foreseeable future.

More than any other major bill proposed in 1993 and 1994, the president's deserves credit for its thoughtful consideration of important options for assuring health care quality.[2] In his address to Congress in September 1993, President Clinton appropriately emphasized: "If we reformed everything else in health care, but failed to preserve and enhance the high quality of our medical care, we will have taken a step backward, not forward. Quality is something that we simply can't leave to chance."[3] Policy analysts and the public would be wise to consider the quality provisions of the president's proposal regardless of the fate that awaits it in Congress. Moreover, as the implementation prospects of this plan come under the microscope, it is worth remembering that a comparable analysis of current efforts to promote quality would yield a lengthy list of inadequacies. Quality assurance poses hard challenges in any health care system, whether it provides universal coverage or not.

States, of course, have long been on the front lines of efforts to promote quality. They serve as educator and gatekeeper for health care providers. In this regard, state universities operate about 60 percent of the 126 medical schools in the United States and enroll a majority of all medical students.[4] State boards license individual medical providers to practice, and they participate in the accreditation process for health care institutions. In administering medicaid programs or in purchasing health insurance for their employees, states often encourage regulation and incentives that shape the processes of care. Their promotion of practice guidelines, utilization review, and profile monitoring exemplifies this attention to process. Although often used primarily in an effort to save money, these tools also directly affect the quality of care delivered. Some states have also built their capacity to monitor and report on the performance of particular institutions and physicians—for example, through studies of the mortality rates of patients being treated by particular providers.

In these and countless other ways, states have focused on the inputs, processes, and outcomes of the medical system to help determine the quality of care available to the citizenry. Hence the view from the states has roots in substantial experience. However, the capacity and commitment of state governments in the medical quality arena vary greatly. Some states take the tasks of quality assurance much more seriously than others, and some are much better equipped than others to contribute to efforts to improve and sustain quality.[5]

Before taking up the implementation issues involved in creating smarter markets, firming up medical science through outcomes research, and creating effective mechanisms for voice, it is important to clarify the goal. What does quality health care mean?

Quality: An Elusive Concept

Of the three legs of health care reform—access, cost, and quality—the last presents the most problems of conceptualization and measurement. A top health care official from Florida captured some of the difficulties when he observed that "I can't tell you what [quality] is, but I know bad quality when I see it."[6] Definitions of quality vary, and grappling with them plunges one into a dense empirical and ethical thicket. Impenetrable underbrush often obscures the causal relationship between medical care and its outcomes. Moreover, people at times differ in their judgments of what desirable outcomes are. For instance, even so obvious an outcome measure as prolonging life becomes questionable under some circumstances.

For present purposes, I follow the lead of the congressional Office of Technology Assessment and define medical care quality as "the degree to which the process of care increases the probability of (desired) outcomes . . . and reduces the probability of undesired outcomes, given the state of medical knowledge."[7] Given this basic definition, medical encounters can be construed as falling along a quality continuum with something like "presidential medicine" at one extreme and "abject quackery" at the other.

Quality, of course, should be distinguished from access. The latter targets the ease with which individuals can obtain medical care. It focuses on whether geographic, financial, or other barriers prevent people from getting treated in the medical care system. Quality, in contrast, focuses on the nature of the experience once they make it through the gates of the system. Quality is also not the same as efficiency; rather, it is the benefit, or output, side of the efficiency ratio (output/cost). To be sure, the quest for greater efficiency in the medical care system can yield greater quality. For example, it can help weed out medical interventions that do nothing to promote desired health outcomes and may even expose patients to greater risk. And more efficient treatment of certain diseases may free up resources that can be redeployed to improve the quality of other medical care. But efforts to promote efficiency do not always yield better quality. Some of the hardest decisions faced by providers and policymakers involve low-benefit, high-cost treatment— expensive care that enhances quality only marginally.

In a perfect world for program monitors and evaluators, assessments of the quality of a medical encounter would depend on careful observations of a provider's skills of diagnosis, prognosis, therapeutic and preventive intervention, and interpersonal communication. These skills would be judged in terms of their relationship to desired outcomes. Monitors would be able to score a representative sample of patient encounters with the medical system. From this sample they could plot the distribution of a population's encounters with the system along a quality continuum. This exercise would put them in a better position to gauge the distributional implications of health care reform: the degree to which some groups of people receive better care than others. Trends over time could also be tracked.

Of course, this world is not so perfect for assessing quality. Calibrating and assembling information on the quality of medical encounters poses staggering methodological problems. If comprehensive health care reform occurs, the politics of its implementation would therefore take place in a milieu where the players cannot keep precise track of the quality score. Various stakeholders would attempt to exploit this uncertainty to their strategic advantage. Because cost is so measurable and quality so amorphous, the political dynamics of program evolution could tilt toward an excessive emphasis on economy at the expense of quality. The proposals discussed in this chapter seek to counter any such tendency.

Smarter Markets

Markets can be a force for quality. Providing ample, repeated opportunities for consumers to choose among plans and specific medical personnel puts these providers under pressure to please the customer by delivering quality care. Depending on the flow of valid comprehensible information about cost, access, and quality, however, medical markets can be "smarter" or "dumber." Since the quality of care is so hard to define and measure, the risk is high that consumers will not possess sufficient information to choose intelligently among providers on this dimension.

Sensitivity to this problem has sparked what some refer to as the "report card movement."[8] Large purchasers of care have become increasingly interested in obtaining comparative data on the quality and other characteristics of different plans. For instance, starting in 1989, several employers and managed-care organizations began work on the Health Plan Employer Data and Information Set (HEDIS). They believed that this would ultimately be a tool for large purchasers to use in judging the relative value (including quality) of competing health plans. In addition, more than thirty states have mandated the development of public domain health data sets that could become the foundation for performance reports. For example, the Pennsylvania Health Care Cost Commission has released comparative hospital data concerning different measures of performance for the fifty-three most common diagnosis-related groups. Sensing the potential relevance of these and other developments, health care reformers of various political stripes have advocated the use of report cards.[9] None, however, surpasses the Clinton plan in its commitment to this tool.

An Ambitious Proposal

The White House Domestic Policy Council sets forth the thrust of the Clinton plan: "Under the Health Security Act, American consumers will benefit from greater access to information, which in turn will further improve quality. They will exercise not only the right to choose doctors, other health providers and health plans, but also the right to make informed choices based on meaningful information about how health plans, health professionals and hospitals perform."[10] Annual performance reports, or report cards, would underpin this effort. Under the Clinton proposal, "each regional alliance shall make available to eligible enrollees information in an easily understood and useful form, that allows such enrollees . . . to make valid comparisons among health plans offered by the alliance." This information on cost, access, and quality is to be available in a brochure, published at least once a year.[11]

A newly created national quality management council would lead the charge to develop quality indicators. Subsumed under a federal national health board, the quality council would consist of fifteen members appointed by the president for three-year staggered terms. The president would designate one of these individuals as the chair. The council would include members from at least five categories of interests—government and corporate purchasers of health care, the health plans, state governments, health care providers, and academic health centers—as well as other experts on quality. Beyond this, the proposed Health Security Act directs the council to reach out to other stakeholders in its deliberations, including three federal bureaucracies: the Agency for Health Care Policy and Research, the National Institutes of Health, and the Health Care Financing Administration. The quality management council would also have to confer with a newly established national quality consortium, consisting of eleven individuals representing academic health centers, schools of public health, and related educational entities. The quality council would depend heavily on the national health board and other federal agencies for staff support.

The lead role assigned to the quality council reflects a desire to collect information in a standard format that would ultimately permit comparison of all regional alliances and plans. The proposal charges the quality council with developing indicators on a wide array of subjects, including access to health care services by consumers; appropriateness of health care services; the outcomes of services and procedures; health promotion; prevention of diseases, disorders, and other health conditions; and consumer satisfaction with care. The Clinton bill also takes pains to specify criteria that should guide the quality council in developing and selecting performance measures. The measures would need to be "reliable and valid," and as a whole, "representative of the range of services" provided to consumers of health care. The indicators would emphasize "significance" by focusing on health conditions that are more prevalent, have higher morbidity and mortality rates, and cost more to treat. If a measure focuses on a process, the quality council would need to understand the relationship of this process to the "health outcome." The outcome measures would have to be ones that providers could affect. In a bow toward recognizing information costs, the selection of indicators would also take into account whether data collection would impose an "undue burden" on plans and providers.

Whenever the quality council determined that "sufficient information and consensus exist," it would recommend to the national health board that it establish goals for performance by health plans and providers. The indicators endorsed by the board would undergird the annual report cards prepared by the alliances and plans. Armed with these reports, the quality council would each year submit to Congress its assessment of the quality of care being achieved across the country.

The Health Security Act would establish a new encounter-based electronic data system to supply the information to satisfy the need for quality indicators. This information system would include data on the patients' clinical encounters with health care providers, enrollment and disenrollment in the health plans, and grievances filed with the alliances. To accomplish this, the national health board would oversee a vast "electronic data network consisting of regional centers that collect, compile, and transmit information." This network would be tested before implementation through demonstration projects. National requirements for medical records would supersede any contrary provisions in state law.

To gain further insight into plan performance, the quality council would "conduct periodic surveys of health care consumers to gather information concerning access to care, use of health services, health outcomes, and patient satisfaction." The Agency for Health Care Policy and Research (AHCPR) would administer the surveys on a "plan-by-plan, state-by-state basis." State officials would have the opportunity to add items beyond those deemed essential by the federal government. At least some of the responses to the surveys would become part of the annual performance reports of the plans.

The efforts to create information-rich, smarter markets does not end with the annual report cards. The alliances would also be responsible for reviewing the plans' marketing materials to ensure that the plans did not distribute misleading information to consumers. The alliance would also make sure that plans did not advertise in only one area of the alliance region in order to attract only preferred customers.

The Perilous Road to Smart Markets

Ultimately, the Clinton effort to make the health care market more aware of quality depends on four processes: the determination of valid indicators of quality by the plans; the collection and analysis of data concerning how well plans meet these criteria; the timely, effective dissemination of this information; and the constructive use of this information by consumers and other key players. As will become evident, none of these processes can be taken for granted.

In all probability, administrative agencies at both the federal and state levels lack the capacity (such as enough competent personnel, funding, and expertise) and in some cases the commitment needed to implement the report card provisions of the Clinton plan. This circumstance in part reflects general limits to the state of the art in quality measurement. The question is not, then, whether the implementation road to smart markets has potholes, for it surely does; the question is whether the road is completely washed out, whether a detour will help, or whether a new destination is needed.

GROPING FOR INDICATORS. Can a sample of currently available indicators yield a collage that accurately conveys to consumers the quality of care offered by the plans? Or will the present unavailability of more important and representative indicators undermine any such effort? The latter scenario seems more likely. As a legislative analyst from California noted: "We have been struggling to measure quality in health care for years. And we have gotten a lot of interesting indicators of a lot of pieces of health care quality with respect to a lot of specific conditions. But we have a mosaic that's very, very sparsely filled in so far."[12]

The sheer technical demands of finding a valid, representative sample of indicators to gauge access, appropriateness, outcomes, health promotion, disease prevention, and customer satisfaction are breathtaking. Selecting certain of the indicators would be particularly hard. Consider outcomes, in some respects the most fundamental measure of provider performance. To present a fair picture, officials could not simply report death rates (or some other outcome) for hospitals and providers for certain procedures. The rates would require risk adjustment, or hospitals and doctors who treated sicker people would almost always look worse on the report cards. The federal government and such states as New York and California have demonstrated that mortality outcome studies can be done. But their experience indicates that progress in developing and presenting this information is better measured in inches than miles.

New York State, for instance, has worked to develop mortality report cards on providers since the late 1980s. A report released by the state Department of Health in December 1993 on death rates from cardiac surgery illustrates the result. The seventeen-page booklet, which the department publicized in the media and promptly distributed to all those requesting copies, presented risk-adjusted mortality rates for coronary artery bypass grafts in thirty-one New York hospitals licensed to perform the procedure. The report also detailed a risk-adjusted mortality rate for each of eighty-seven surgeons who had performed at least 200 such operations in the same hospital from 1990 through 1992. The report uncovered one hospital with a significantly lower mortality rate and one with a significantly higher number. Out of the eighty-seven surgeons, eight had a risk-adjusted mortality rate significantly greater than the statewide figure and four had rates significantly less than this norm.[13]

New York's analytic achievement deserves praise but needs to be kept in perspective. It took ample resources and several iterations to score hospitals and providers on just this one procedure. By the time the report came out, its information was already somewhat dated. Moreover, for all their complexity, mortality studies of this kind tend to be easier to do than analyses focused on the outcomes of care that can improve health but is not a life-or-death matter.

As if these technical difficulties were not sufficient, the political problem of building administrative consensus on quality indicators would also loom very large. The players involved would bring sharply contrasting perspectives to the task. For instance, the national quality management council and several federal agencies might well push hard to develop a probing, valid report card. Plans and providers, however, would enter the negotiation with an acute desire to reduce their own costs of collecting the information. Providers would also be concerned about selecting indicators for which they could get a good score and that would not slight the more subtle side of medical care.

Some state officials have had firsthand experience with how protracted a challenge reaching agreement on indicators can be. Again New York State provides an example. Officials in the state Department of Health wanted to develop a handful of measures for health maintenance organizations (HMOs) focused on preventive care, such as prenatal visits, immunizations, and mammographies. Negotiations with the HMOs initially focused on getting one indicator for immunizations. Much to the frustration of New York officials, it took five months to reach agreement on this one measure, a pace that an HMO official thought was "exceptionally fast." Extrapolating to the annual performance reports called for by the Clinton plan, a top executive in the New York Department of Health concluded, "At that rate, we will get to 50 indicators [by] the time none of us are around to appreciate it."[14]

Advocates for those suffering from particular diseases would add to the complexity of reaching consensus. As one state official put it, "I am afraid that when the feds start laying on a list of things that we have to measure, there is going to be that disease of the month syndrome. . . . You can come up with a very fantastical list, and nobody wants to be left off."[15] Those whose diseases were not listed on the report card promulgated by the national health board would probably attack the tool as invalid and might bring suit in court. Mustering scientific claims for the validity of report cards would not be easy for defenders, given the gross limits to knowledge about how to develop valid summary measures of the quality of medical care. The report card could come to reflect the political muscle of various groups of disease advocates as much as it did more scientific assessments of quality.

Once officials selected the indicators, plans would be tempted to adjust their methods of providing care to do well on the report cards, regardless of the implications for other important medical objectives. A legislative analyst from California cut to the crux of this matter when he predicted probable plan reactions to poor performance on such indicators as immunizations and Pap smears. He noted that plans would respond to this feedback by doing more of both procedures. But "what trade-offs does the plan do to direct the resources toward immunizations?" Does it increase Pap smears "at the price of having less effective follow-up when the results come in?" Given these dynamics, he worried about "focusing on specific narrow indicators."[16]

MINING AND ASSAYING INFORMATION. Reaching agreement on quality indicators would be only the first step. Collecting and analyzing the data called for by the indicators would also present challenges. The plans and providers would bear much of the costs of furnishing the information needed for report cards. They would be concerned that the data they submitted would not damage them in the competition for enrollees. Patient preferences for the confidentiality of medical records could also fuel concern. Resistance and delay seem likely. In this regard, an official in the New York Department of Social Services noted that "we should anticipate a substantial amount of conflict between the plans and the regional alliances regarding information sharing. . . . The technology is there to do it, [but] it will be very difficult to get the information in the form you want."[17] A top health official from another state conveyed a similar concern when she observed that her "state has all the authority in the world to say, 'Give us that data and give it to us right this minute.' And yet there is a tremendous amount of reluctance by the plans and the hospitals as well as the docs to give us that data."[18]

Verifying the accuracy of the data submitted by the plans would also take time and effort. The transmitted information would probably contain many errors and require substantial "scrubbing." For instance, when officials in the New York Department of Health collected basic data for the outcomes study focused on coronary artery bypass grafts, the reports submitted by hospitals often contained basic mistakes about patients' sex and whether they were dead or alive. To obtain enough data just to report periodically on the outcomes of this one procedure, the health department had to devote three full-time-equivalent employees to the task each year.[19]

Not all the data related to the quality indicators would be so hard to collect and scrub. Matters would improve over time as the electronic data system matured. But even then the costs of obtaining, cleaning, and analyzing information would be formidable.

DISSEMINATION AND USE. Given the complexities of agreeing on indicators and assembling the needed information, report cards (at least sophisticated versions of them) would be slow in reaching an alliance's population. As a New York official predicted, "People are going to be making choices well ahead of when report cards are really going to be available in any meaningful way."[20] Fear of litigation could fuel this tardiness, since the alliances would bear liability for any incorrect or misleading information that damaged the reputation of particular plans or providers.

The alliances would also need to work hard to format and design user-friendly report cards and to distribute them widely. The degree to which individuals would use the cards as a factor in their choices of plans and providers remains an open question. Clearly, however, the alliances would encounter an uphill battle to get certain segments of the population, such as those who are illiterate or do not speak English well, to use them. As one state official emphasized, these individuals would have less meaningful "opportunity to vote with their feet." Efforts by the states to overcome the information deficits faced by the less advantaged could well drive up administrative costs.[21]

Assessment and Alternatives

Implementing the requirements for valid report cards would be impossible in the time frame envisioned by the proposed Health Security Act. To be sure, administrators could eventually iron out some of the problems. Implementation analysis will not serve policy debate well if it becomes excessively preoccupied with short-term start-up costs and issues. Even so, using report cards to make markets smarter about quality presents a major challenge that would not be easily met in the foreseeable future.

Given this problem, one approach is to affirm that report cards (or the quality component of them) are simply not worth the trouble, that comprehensive health care reform packages should not mandate them. Such an approach would hardly be the death knell for quality. Other forces exist to prod the medical care system toward quality, the education and professional commitments of health care personnel being first and foremost. Nor from a market perspective should it be assumed that people respond only to price in the absence of crisp quality indicators. In fact, some analysis suggests that patients at times use higher prices as a proxy for quality. More commonly, however, people have ways of judging quality that, although far from ideal, are certainly not far-fetched. Many studies indicate that in selecting providers people rely heavily on word of mouth, seeking the advice of friends and relatives.[22] This advice need not be bad. Moreover, people gain experience with providers, form judgments, and often vote with their feet if they become dissatisfied with care. Preserving an attractive menu of health plans so that consumers have a viable exit option would be more important than developing finely honed report cards.

A second, probably more desirable, possibility is to mandate report cards but stress a more modest, deregulated, decentralized, phased-in approach than that embodied in the Clinton health plan. Using this approach, the best would not become the enemy of the good. Although report cards cannot present a complete quality picture, they can assist consumers when kept in perspective as one among many possible sources of pertinent information about quality.[23] Scorecards can temper the tendency of plans to stress economy at the expense of quality. Some meaningful data can be collected for report cards without enormous expense (such as the numbers of those who file valid complaints against the plan or responses to customer surveys). Nor would all consumers need to use the performance reports to make them worthwhile. Economists stress that the number of expert buyers in many markets tends to be small, but that this group of knowledgeable consumers can often be a potent enough force to tip the market toward an emphasis on quality.[24]

In encouraging report cards, however, the national government should not bite off more than it can chew at an early point. With all the other implementation problems the federal government would face in getting a national health care program off the ground, it should at a minimum postpone detailed, central direction of the report card initiative. It should instead mandate that all plans produce these cards annually, sketch some general criteria, and then allow the states, the alliances, and the plans to negotiate the specifics.

The federal government could retain the ultimate authority over the report cards through its role in reviewing and approving the quality component of state plans. It should steadily apply pressure to ensure greater uniformity in medical record-keeping. It could offer technical assistance by striving to develop indicators of quality and a model report card, which states might choose to adopt. As the federal government's information systems improved over time and it won some victories on other important fronts, federal officials could turn their attention to racheting up standards for the report cards through the Federal Register and other vehicles. In the meantime, federal agencies would diffuse conflict to the states. They would also learn more about what works and what does not by assessing variation in state approaches to report cards.

Outcomes Research and Practice Guidelines

The pursuit of quality under comprehensive health care reform also intersects with initiatives to improve the scientific basis of medicine and the promulgation of practice guidelines.[25] Medicine, as one physician has noted, "is a curious mixture of a highly effective technology interspersed with islands of dogma, empiricism, conventional wisdom, and at times, superstition."[26] The link between medical intervention and patient outcomes is often highly uncertain. Another physician summed it up as follows:

It should be disturbing to us as a profession that we have so few outcomes data and use so few in our practices. Most of us do not learn enough in our training to collect or analyze our own data or interpret consistently the work of others. Early in our training, however, we learn to live and deal with uncertainty. . . . We clearly have a bias toward action. . . . We learn to enjoy playing the game of medical care without hard evidence, and the outcome—often unknown in statistical terms—is of secondary importance to the process.[27]

Research that beams light on the outcomes of medical intervention can provide a better foundation for practice guidelines. These guidelines can in turn promote quality and efficiency by identifying "best practice." Health care reformers believe that the guidelines can buttress the ability of medical providers to resist pressures for worthless or low-benefit, high-cost care. They can help protect doctors against claims of medical malpractice.

One variant of outcomes research began to attract considerable attention in Congress in the 1980s. Policy entrepreneurs, led by John Wennberg of the Dartmouth College Medical School, dramatized the shaky empirical base of medical science by underscoring the great variations in treatment of the same disease from one area of the country to the next. For instance, Wennberg noted that patients being treated for angina in New Haven were more than twice as likely as their counterparts in Boston to undergo surgery. Providers in Boston tended to rely more on angioplasty or drugs. Variations like this immediately prompt the question: Which practices produce better outcomes and hence higher-quality care? Wennberg and his associates promised Congress that evaluative research targeted on variation in medical practice could provide much of the answer. He urged that funding for this form of outcomes research be "on par" with that devoted to traditional biomedical science.[28] Advocates for outcomes research won a partial victory when the Omnibus Budget Reconciliation Act of 1989 created the federal Agency for Health Care Policy and Research. The funding of outcomes research and the promulgation of practice guidelines became a core mission of the new agency.[29]

AHCPR joined a highly decentralized, pluralistic structure for issuing practice guidelines. These guidelines come in many forms (from three-page documents to book-length treatises) and emanate from a number of private and public entities, including medical societies, insurance companies, hospitals, the Institute of Medicine of the National Academy of Sciences, medicare and medicaid, and the National Institutes of Health. These guidelines spring from diverse methodologies, and most do not rest on the kind of outcomes research advocated by Wennberg.[30]

For comprehensive health care reformers, outcomes research and practice guidelines come down to two key scenarios. The first involves using the tools primarily as a vehicle for educating physicians and creating smarter markets. In this vein, government could stimulate research and alert medical providers and quality-conscious consumers to the latest findings and practice protocols. Equipped with better knowledge and, possibly, feeling greater market pressures to achieve efficiency, providers and patients would presumably be less inclined to pursue worthless or low-benefit, high-cost care.

Under the second scenario, government would transform guidelines into regulation. Best or appropriate practice would thereby become codified into law and administrative edict. Armed with better evidence, government would assume a more central role in developing guidelines, picking among them, legitimating them, and enforcing them. Of course, a substantial amount of regulation exists in the current medical system. Under the banners of economy, efficiency, and (to a more limited degree) quality assurance, those paying the bills for medical care employ utilization review, profile monitoring, and other tools to make judgments about the appropriateness of the care delivered to their enrollees.[31]

They often refuse to pay for "inappropriate" care. Under this second scenario, an initiative on behalf of outcomes research and practice guidelines would seek to centralize and rationalize this existing patchwork of regulation.

The Clinton Approach: Both Scenarios

In endorsing outcomes research and practice protocols, the Clinton proposal contains elements of both the educational and regulatory scenarios. In part, the Clinton administration views outcomes research and practice guidelines as vehicles for regulatory relief. In this vein, it promises that "the Health Security Act will replace the outmoded system for measuring quality in practice today, where government bureaucrats and insurance companies second-guess decisions made by doctors and their patients. . . . Focusing on results will reduce the paperwork and micromanagement that strangle doctors, nurses, hospitals, and clinics. It frees health professionals from intrusive insurance companies and bureaucrats."[32] As a sign of its commitment to this objective, the Health Security Act proposes to eliminate the federally funded Peer Review Organizations (PROs).[33]

In tossing out one administrative structure, the Clinton plan promises to create another less exclusively focused on regulation. The national quality management council would establish priorities for AHCPR, that among other things, "would emphasize research involving medical conditions to which there is the highest level of uncertainty concerning treatment and the widest variation in practice patterns." The Clinton bill calls for the quality council to direct AHCPR "to develop and periodically review and update clinically relevant guidelines that may be used by health care providers to assist in determining how diseases, disorders, and other health conditions can most effectively and appropriately be prevented, diagnosed, treated, and managed clinically." In this and other ways, the quality council would be a leader in disseminating information "documenting clinically ineffective treatments and procedures."[34] The research conducted would draw on the electronic clinical encounter records that the health plans would presumably establish in response to other provisions of the Health Security Act.

The Clinton plan also would create regional professional foundations to assist in the research and educational effort related to quality. These foundations would be the offspring of a national quality consortium (an eleven-member group of university representatives appointed by the national health board). The foundations would include at least one academic health center as well as other stakeholders (such as health plans, medical providers, and alliances). With advice from the quality consortium, the national health board would determine the geographic area to be included in each region. In addition "to applying for and conducting" outcomes research, the foundations would develop programs in lifetime learning for health professionals. They would disseminate information about successful quality improvement programs, practice guidelines, and research findings and would develop patient education systems.[35]

While these elements emphasize the educational scenario, the Clinton proposal keeps the regulatory club in reserve. Title I of the Health Security Act gives the national health board the authority to promulgate regulations concerning whether "an item or service" is "medically necessary or appropriate."[36] This could be an opening for cementing practice guidelines into the federal code.

Implementation: Efficiency over Quality?

At least three clusters of problems would complicate efforts to implement the Clinton plan: creating another layer of institutions, sustaining an adequate funding base for guidelines based on outcomes research, and surmounting conflict over the substance and regulatory weight of the guidelines.

The Health Security Act calls for creation of new institutions at a time when the national health board and national quality management council would already face overload. The board would have to define appropriate geographic boundaries for the new regional professional foundations and oversee their assembly in consultation with other advisory councils. Transaction costs would be high, and conflict as well as delay seem likely.

These institutional difficulties need not automatically derail outcomes research and practice guidelines, however. An analytic infrastructure (AHCPR, other federal agencies, think tanks, universities) currently exists to pursue research and disseminate information on these subjects. Progress could be made even in the absence of the regional professional foundations and the electronic data system for medical encounters. In some respects, the key implementation question revolves less around the institutional capacity for outcomes research than the willingness of Congress to stay the course in funding it.

Proponents of outcomes research and practice guidelines will not have an easy time competing for federal research dollars. Powerful constituencies supported by favorable public opinion constantly urge Congress to discover new ways to cure diseases. In contrast, outcomes research appeals more to policy wonks interested in the more subtle pursuit of quality and efficiency. Given these dynamics, it is no accident that the budget for AHCPR in fiscal 1994 amounted to $154 million while the appropriation for the National Institutes of Health was roughly $11 billion, about seventy times more.[37]

Whether outcomes research succeeds in attracting more resources depends in large part on whether it lives up to its billing as a way to save money. Proponents of this research have used cost cutting as a major selling point. For instance, two students of variation in medical practice indicate that if outcomes research finds that the lower end of the range of variation represents appropriate care, "thirty percent to fifty percent of the nation's health bill might be said to consist of expenditures on care that produces little or no demonstrable health benefit."[38] Statements like this have built expectations to very high levels, as exemplified by the experience of a medicaid director in Florida:

> Our health reform agency last year was preaching to our legislature how practice parameters could save 20 to 30 percent. . . . The chairman of the Senate Health Committee call[ed] me into his office and [said], "Gary, we are getting ready to do practice parameters. How much money can I cut out of the medicaid budget?" . . . I had a difficult time explaining that it didn't work that way; . . . I didn't quite know how to take . . . the practice parameter on incontinence and translate that into medical cost savings.

Many physicians do not believe that studies of variation in medical practice will consistently point to practice guidelines that save money if researchers truly let the chips fall where they may.[40] At times, doing more, rather than less, serves quality. To the degree that this proves true, the willingness of lawmakers to fund outcomes research may well evaporate.

Even if appropriations for outcomes research are ample, the path to practice guidelines will not be smooth. At its best, research on practice variations cannot eradicate all sources of conflict about appropriate medical practice. Such research seldom eliminates all uncertainty about the efficacy of certain medical interventions; in addition, guidelines are about efficiency as well as quality. Guidelines serve both quality and efficiency when they help stamp out treatments that do nothing to promote health or even do harm. They mainly serve efficiency when they wage war on low-benefit, high-cost care. Proceeding with low-benefit care on the remote chance it will help is more attractive to physicians and patients than to those stuck with picking up the tab for such care.

In the face of empirical uncertainty and the tension between quality and efficiency, forging consensus on practice guidelines and ensuring compliance with them will often be politically difficult. Efforts to promulgate guidelines on mammograms provide a particularly dramatic example. In late 1993 the National Cancer Institute changed its advisory guidelines for mammography screening and recommended that women aged 40 to 49 no longer have mammograms on a regular basis to detect cancer. Among other things, the institute reported that the test did not result in reduced mortality for women who lacked symptoms of the disease. In response to this action, eighteen groups outside government, including the American Cancer Society and the American Medical Association, encouraged women in that age group to ignore the new guidelines and continue to seek mammograms. They argued that the guideline changes were not based on definitive evidence, would confuse women, and would threaten insurer and government reimbursement for the procedures. A Senate subcommittee subsequently grilled and criticized federal health officials for issuing the new guideline.

Guidelines on mammograms obviously press more political hot buttons than would practice parameters targeted at many other medical interventions. Yet David Eddy, a leading proponent of guidelines and a member of the Clinton health team, saw the mammogram issue as a test case. "If we yield every time there's a constituency that can make an emotional argument for coverage of something that is not supported by actual evidence, then we will have a chaotic, expensive and inefficient health care system in this country."[41] There would probably be many such "emotional" arguments as government issued more guidelines. The conflict generated by the guidelines would intensify to the degree that they emphasize efficiency over quality concerns, and that government attempts to write the practice parameters into law or administrative regulation.

Once officials managed to issue a given set of practice guidelines, they could not rest easy. Compliance would be far from automatic. Moreover, the rapid pace of technological change in medicine makes guideline development a Sisyphean task; many practice protocols would require constant updating, bringing a new round of conflict. Even in the absence of medical breakthroughs, new evidence about the outcomes of existing treatments would occasionally surface and in some cases cast doubt about the validity of prior guidelines. Federal officials would then need to revise these protocols. Such error correction would often trigger intense negative publicity, especially if the federal government had written the previous guidelines into official regulation. Under this circumstance, federal agencies could come under searing attack for having damaged the health of the populace.

Federal Leadership, not Centralized Regulation

National health care reform can benefit from encouraging outcomes research and practice guidelines. To be sure, the effect of these efforts on the quality of medical care or the efficiency with which it gets delivered would probably not be huge. But on the margins, this quest for better medical knowledge and practice can help.

It falls naturally to the national government to assume a major leadership role in sponsoring and encouraging research on the outcomes of variations in medical practice. As with biomedical research, the federal government has a comparative advantage over most states as a sponsor and initiator. Moreover, some state officials hope that the federal government would take the heat for issuing practice guidelines since it would help them to alter medical practice in their own states. All of this is not, of course, to suggest that states should play no role. Some states, such as Maine, have demonstrated initiative in the area.[42] But, as the Clinton plan recognizes, the federal government can appropriately serve as a major engine for reform in this sphere.

In encouraging outcomes research and practice guidelines, however, those committed to comprehensive health care reform should do their utmost to avoid central regulation and administrative complexity. The federal government should consider putting guidelines into law or administrative regulation only as a last resort, and perhaps not even then. Transforming guidelines into administrative regulation (via the national health board, under the Clinton plan) would immerse the federal government in conflict and litigation and subject it to much criticism. Moreover, formalizing guidelines into regulation and keeping them current requires a major expenditure of money, time, and effort. Letting guidelines be guidelines rather than regulation carries the political advantage of diffusing conflict and hard decisions to plans and providers, who are on the front lines of the medical system.

Although health plans would not have to comply with the practice guidelines in the absence of law or regulation, they would have some incentive to do so, especially if they were subject to market competition or caps on their revenues. By using the guidelines to reject worthless or low-benefit, high-cost care, they could better compete with other plans in holding costs down. The plans, rather than government, would place pressure on physicians to pay attention to the practice protocols. Nor could the plans ignore guidelines that called for more expensive procedures: failure to comply might expose them to malpractice litigation and the loss of their enrollees to other plans.

Of course, the federal government should have the authority to define the basic benefit package available to citizens under national health care. In this role, it would occasionally need to make Solomonic judgments as to whether plans should provide certain services, such as those emanating from new technologies that show promise but have not been thoroughly tested. But issuing laws or regulations embodying general decisions on benefits (such as coverage for mammograms) is a far cry from doing the same for detailed practice guidelines (such as precise specification of when mammograms should be employed). To its credit, the federal government has avoided the top-down promulgation of practice protocols in its own medicare program. Decisions on what constitutes appropriate care remain substantially decentralized to peer review organizations, providers, and insurance carriers in different regions of the country.[43]

National health care reformers should also try to avoid adding to administrative complexity as they promote outcomes research and practice protocols. The educational and research functions to be performed by the regional professional foundations under the Clinton plan are commendable, but it is far from clear that the federal government should establish a whole new set of institutions and geographic boundaries. If the foundations are needed at all, it would be easier to organize them on a state-by-state basis. Academic health centers could still constitute

the heart of the foundations. Properly structured incentives could encourage states to enter into compacts with each other on projects better
conducted across state boundaries.

Consumer Voice

Comprehensive health care reform should also take into account the
potential and limits of mechanisms for consumer voice as a vehicle for
quality assurance. Obviously, elementary norms of due process imply
that those enrolled in plans must be able to take their grievances somewhere for resolution. Efforts to use consumer sentiment to assess and
promote quality go beyond this, however.

The attractiveness of mechanisms for voice depends in part on the
capacity of patients to judge quality. Some evidence casts doubt on
the validity and reliability of consumer judgment. For instance, one
analysis indicates that seven to eight times as many patients suffered
injury from negligence as the number who filed malpractice claims.
Yet it also appears that 85 percent of malpractice suits occur in cases
where there was no negligence or marked departure from norms of
quality care.[44]

On balance, however, existing research tends to support the view
that patients can provide valuable information about quality. They tend
to be the only readily available source of information about the interpersonal dimension of care. The evidence suggests that patient ratings
of this dimension are comparable to those reached by a panel of experts
reviewing the same interaction. Various studies indicate that providers
whose patients do not rate them positively on interpersonal manner and
skills tend to be less knowledgeable about their patients. Consumers
can even cast some light on the technical quality of care. To be sure,
some evidence suggests that patient ratings of this dimension tend to
be higher than assessments by physicians. And the evidence is mixed
on whether patients tend to give the technical quality of care higher
ratings simply if they receive more services. But at least for some
conditions, patient ratings appear to be quite sensitive to documented
variations in the technical quality of health care.[45]

Evidence like this points to the wisdom of devising institutions to
solicit consumer voice. This exercise requires careful calibration. If
institutions promise great rewards to patients for documenting failure
in physician performance (for example, through malpractice suits), qual-

ity and efficiency can be threatened by encouraging physicians to pursue defensive medicine to a fault.

Surveys, Ombudsmen, and Malpractice

The Clinton plan goes to great lengths to create mechanisms for consumer voice.[46] As already discussed, it aggressively seeks to learn the views of consumers by requiring the national quality management council, in concert with federal agencies, to conduct periodic consumer surveys on a "plan-by-plan, state-by-state basis." These surveys would gauge patient satisfaction and probe specific perceptions of access and quality.

The Clinton plan also creates institutions for handling complaints. All health plans would establish grievance procedures for enrollees. Each regional alliance would also establish and maintain an ombudsman office to assist consumers. To help cover the costs of these offices, states would have the option of permitting those enrolled to designate one dollar of each premium to support the alliance ombudsman.

The Health Security Act tackles malpractice reform through three steps. First, it seeks to reduce the role of the courts by requiring each regional and corporate plan to adopt one of three alternative dispute resolution systems: arbitration, mediation, or "a process under which parties are required to make early offers of settlement."[47] The national health board would define and specify these alternatives through administrative regulation. Only after a dissatisfied patient exhausted the possibility of remedy through this system could he or she bring suit in court.

Second, the Clinton plan seeks to reduce the financial incentives to go to court. It allows courts to impose sanctions and costs on plaintiffs if their complaints are false; it limits attorneys' contingency fees in such cases to no more than one-third of the overall settlement amount; and it allows for the settlement to be reduced by the amount of damages a plaintiff receives from certain other sources, such as private disability programs. These reform provisions would preempt state laws to the extent they were inconsistent with these limitations, but would not interfere with state initiatives that went further in curtailing the liability of medical providers for malpractice.[48]

Third, the Clinton plan proposes two demonstration projects related to malpractice liability. One would examine whether substituting mal-

practice liability of the health plan as a collectivity for the personal
liability of the physician "will result in improvements in the quality of
care provided . . . , reductions in defensive medical practices, and better
risk management."[49] Another calls upon the secretary of Health and
Human Services to provide funds to one or more states to determine the
effect of applying practice guidelines in the resolution of medical malpractice actions. To be eligible for the grant, the state would have to
agree that a physician's adherence to appropriate practice guidelines
would constitute a complete legal defense against an allegation of negligence.

Implementation for a Price

None of the mechanisms for consumer voice built into the Clinton
plan fly in the face of implementation reality. However, they assume
adequate funding and staffing levels. Given the propensity of American
politics to produce many more statutory requirements than agencies
have the resources to carry out, one cannot assume this administrative
capacity would be present.

The federal government, especially through its National Center for
Health Statistics, has a credible track record in performing high-quality
surveys tapping consumer perceptions of their health and the medical
system.[50] The Clinton plan would greatly increase the demands on the
center or other survey agencies. It would require them to go beyond
national surveys and develop a credible methodology for stratified sam-
pling at the state and plan levels. It would force them to develop new
measures related to quality (such as consumer satisfaction). Accomplishing these and related tasks would require time and much effort; the
federal government would have to solicit the cooperation of state officials
and plans (for example, by obtaining lists of those enrolled in the plans).
But, given adequate funding, federal officials could rely on a highly
sophisticated analytic infrastructure to design and conduct the surveys.
They would not be starting from scratch.

Capacity concerns also apply to other provisions of the Clinton plan.
Assuming the alliances can be assembled in the first place, there is
nothing intrinsically intractable about the implementation issues that
either the ombudsman or malpractice system would pose. Again, however, money is the key. Underfunded ombudsmen would mean 800
numbers that do not get answered and complaints that take "forever"

to process. Any tendency toward penury would probably be less evident in the case of the alternative dispute resolution systems for malpractice cases. Both the plans and providers would have a stake in seeing them succeed since investment in these systems could subsequently save them money.

Helpful on the Margins

Mechanisms for consumer voice are not panaceas for assuring quality, but they can help. Patients frequently possess important insights about quality. Although many would not file complaints when they received poor care, consumer surveys are a way to reach beyond this reluctance and tap their perspectives. Since pressures to contain costs would probably be acute under a comprehensive reform plan, sensitivity to consumer concerns can help keep quality from being placed on the back burner.

The utility of mechanisms for voice depends not only on consumer perceptiveness concerning quality but on whether the mechanisms stimulate providers to sustain and improve good medical practice. Both federal and state governments have important roles to play in making sure this occurs. Given its strong track record with health care surveys, the federal government should take the lead in this sphere. Just as the federal government monitors economic indicators (such as unemployment or inflation rates), it can appropriately take center stage in developing survey data related to the quality of care. Federal agencies can provide Congress and state officials with periodic quality reports based on state-by-state surveys. Although these would not be definitive assessments of quality, they would provide useful feedback and prod stakeholders to seek improvements.

Working together, federal and state governments can also assess whether surveys conducted on a plan-by-plan basis could be implemented at reasonable cost. If so, responses to surveys could contribute to smarter markets by becoming part of the report cards for each plan. States could also publish data on valid complaints or malpractice claims for each plan. They could take into account the frequency and severity of valid complaints against practitioners in their licensure and accreditation decisions. Simultaneously, states can work for malpractice reforms that would keep physicians from being so sensitive to consumer voice as to fuel ineffective and inefficient care.

Conclusion

It remains an open question whether quality will be sacrificed to access and cost containment under comprehensive health care reform. As a New York State official observed, much depends on the validity of "the notion that there is 20 to 30 percent excess medical practice that is not adding to quality." Much also depends on whether comprehensive reform can prune other sources of waste in the current medical system (such as the huge overhead costs imposed by the multiplicity of insurance companies and plans). Focusing on the Clinton plan, which would limit premium growth, the New York administrator cautioned that the alliances are "going to be faced [with] the pressure of trying to live within some rate of growth of spending that has never been achieved before." He questioned whether quality could be maintained "when the fiscal pressures are so significant."[51]

If comprehensive reform succeeded in reducing providers' revenues, providers would face pressures to become salespersons for doing less. Some of this effort would target worthless or low-benefit, high-cost care. But, pushed to an extreme, the pressures would resemble those in the British health care system. Trained to treat illness, British doctors find themselves unable to provide all the medical care that might benefit their patients. In response, as Henry J. Aaron and William B. Schwartz note, British "doctors gradually redefine standards of care so that they can escape the constant recognition that financial limits compel them to do less than their best. By various means, physicians and other health care providers try to make the denial of care seem routine or optimal."[52] Tight fiscal constraints (as well as regulatory initiatives) could also endanger quality by retarding the development of new technologies and drugs. Rapid technological innovation accounts for much of the growth in medical expenditures.[53]

It remains far from clear, of course, that the politics of implementation and program evolution under comprehensive health care reform would in fact impose severe financial restraints on the medical system. Powerful constituencies—physicians, advocates for cures of various diseases, industries involved in medical technology and drugs, patients— would strongly resist draconian cuts. For example, policymakers have already begun discussion of how to ensure the continued flow of funding to the National Institutes of Health (NIH) under health care reform.[54] A major sponsor of medical research, NIH has traditionally fared well in Washington's budget processes. Moreover, even if pressures to contain costs intensify, the result might well be diminished access to care for some people rather than a general decline in the quality of medical encounters. If expenses rose too steeply for government and employers under a national health plan, policymakers would be tempted to reduce the scope of the benefit package or impose more deductibles and copayments on patients. If these cuts occur, more affluent citizens would tend to purchase supplemental policies. The poor would be less likely to do so. Thus class-based access to medical care would reassert itself. Still, the risk to quality posed by cost containment initiatives under comprehensive health care reform is sufficient that issues of quality assurance deserve careful consideration. This analysis suggests that health care reformers should keep six general propositions in mind.

First, the best hope for quality is redundancy: many mechanisms focused on quality, no one of which may have great effect but which as a whole can help keep the medical system on its toes. The three clusters of tools discussed here—smarter markets through report cards, practice guidelines based on outcomes research, and mechanisms for consumer voice—need to be judged in this context. It would be utter folly to see any of the three as the magic elixir of quality assurance. Even if implemented, none of them would have a major effect on the quality of care, at least over the short term. Comprehensive health care reform that included none of the three elements might still improve the quality of care for large segments of the population. However, the three approaches can be a useful addition to the arsenal of mechanisms aimed at promoting quality (along with such measures as licensure, accreditation, medical school education and socialization, and biomedical research). The Clinton administration deserves much credit for having elevated the three approaches to a more central position on the policy agenda.

Whether report cards, practice guidelines, or mechanisms for voice will add to or subtract from existing quality assurance efforts depends largely on their implementation. Much depends on the capacities and commitments of critical players at the state and federal levels as well as the chemistry of their interaction, in particular, the extent of cooperation and conflict. Policies that take these implementation issues into account stand a fighting chance of success.

Second, assessments of the relative capacity and commitment of different levels of government should in part guide judgments about the appropriate division of labor in programs to assure quality. In some areas, the federal government has a comparative advantage over the states. Having generally carved out a niche as a major sponsor of research and development, the national government can appropriately take the lead in spurring research on outcomes and practice protocols. Drawing on pertinent experience and substantial expertise, it can also direct and administer the consumer surveys. In other areas, such as malpractice, federal officials know enough to set basic floors and then welcome state efforts to rise above them. But in other spheres, such as the development of valid report cards, the federal government has less comparative advantage and should probably defer to the states.

Third, questions of the division of labor also revolve around political criteria related to how much and where conflict should occur in the political system. Which level of government can and should take the heat? State officials at times have expressed the hope that the federal government would issue practice guidelines because they wanted to avoid the ensuing controversy. State administrators often find it useful to blame the "feds" for initiatives they really want to pursue anyway. But there are limits to the political pounding that the federal government can take. At times, its credibility is better served by diffusing conflict rather than focusing it toward Washington. The transformation of practice guidelines into law or administrative regulation stands out as an issue for the federal government to avoid. As Lawrence D. Brown has noted, most Western democracies try to regulate health care budgets and not to micromanage the specific delivery of care.[55] Although no doubt difficult to apply in the United States, this practice deserves emulation. Decisions on how to apply practice guidelines are best left to plans and providers. A few state governments may find it in their interest to undertake this task. But the federal government should consider writing practice protocols into law or regulation only if other cost containment measures fail and no other viable alternatives present themselves.

Fourth, in some instances a decentralized, deregulated, phased-in approach to quality assurance would allow the federal government to learn from various state experiences. For example, the federal government does not know how to create a valid definitive performance report card. At best, the report cards are likely to shed partial light on quality. By asking states to come up with performance reports that provide at least some useful information, the federal government not only escapes administrative overload and conflict, it opens the door to experimentation and learning.

Fifth, reliance on the states, or at least respecting state boundaries, can reduce administrative fragmentation and complexity. Over the years, American health care reformers have delighted in defining new geographic boundaries for certain health care functions and creating new regional institutions to serve them. To the degree that these initiatives ignore state boundaries, however, administrative complexities increase and accountability becomes ever more blurred. In the case of the Clinton plan, for instance, it would probably be better to establish professional foundations for research and education related to practice guidelines on a state-by-state basis rather than create whole new territories for them. If necessary, incentives could be provided for interstate cooperation.

Sixth, any discussion of assuring quality under comprehensive health care reform also needs to consider the risk involved in sticking with the status quo. If the United States forgoes major policy change and continues on its present course, medical prices will probably continue to rise sharply and growing numbers of Americans will be without adequate health insurance. This development would not only create barriers to access, it would also encourage plans and physicians to cut corners on quality in treating those who could not pay the full bill. These consequences may well pose a greater threat to the health of the populace than any quality problems associated with comprehensive reform.

In sum, proponents of quality assurance under comprehensive health care reform cannot escape the challenge of implementing programs through the federal system. This challenge would be significant but, sensibly approached, far from insurmountable.

5 ||| Reform and the Medical Work Force: Choices and Challenges

Michael S. Sparer

THE CLINTON health care reform proposal seeks to make significant changes in both the composition and the practice patterns of America's medical work force.[1] The goals are to produce more generalists (and fewer specialists) and to encourage more health care professionals of all types to practice in medically underserved communities.[2] Although this effort receives relatively little public attention, Clinton administration officials consider it a critical component of the broader agenda of cost containment and universal coverage.[3] Why is there a connection? First, the nation has too many medical specialists, who run up costs by overtesting and overtreating.[4] Second, the uninsured need access to a system of good quality primary care, which simply does not exist in too many communities. And third, generalist providers are the administrative linchpin of any managed-care system, providing patients with necessary primary care and guiding them away from unnecessary specialty treatment.

The plan delegates to the federal government responsibility for altering the composition of the nation's medical work force. The plan would create a national institute for health care work force development, which would make recommendations on medical work force needs and priorities. Moreover, and more important, by 1998 a new national council on graduate medical education would impose a cap on the total number of medical residents; allocate the number of residencies in each medical specialty; and ensure that 55 percent of all new residents are trained as generalists.[5]

The plan is less clear, however, about how government (at any level) is to encourage more providers to practice in medically underserved communities. There is, instead, a hodgepodge of provisions to improve access: some address the work force problem directly (by providing economic incentives for health professionals to practice in underserved communities); others suggest indirect solutions (such as expanding the institutional settings for primary care in the hope that if facilities are built providers will come); and still others delegate the problem to state and local governments (for example, requiring that states be the ultimate guarantor of adequate access).

For example, the plan would provide federal funds to develop and implement a host of relatively small programs to recruit minority providers, train nonphysician providers (such as nurse-practitioners and physician assistants), and encourage health professionals of all types to work in indigent communities. Federal funds also would be available for medically underserved communities that develop or expand institutional settings for primary care providers (such as school health clinics).[6] Health alliances can offer financial inducements to health plans to encourage them to expand into medically underserved communities.[7] Health plans must contract, for at least five years, with "essential community providers" (thus providing at least some protection to the medical safety net now in place). And states must themselves somehow ensure that all consumers have access to a choice of good health plans.[8]

The Clinton plan represents an ambitious and important effort to recast federal policy away from encouraging institution-based specialty care and toward community-based generalist care. This effort is particularly noteworthy because it challenges fifty years of federal health policy and does so in an intelligent and interesting way. Given this context, before discussing the specifics of the Clinton plan, I review briefly how fifty years of federal health policy has shaped the current medical work force.

Fifty Years of Federal Policies

Federal policy has shaped the U.S. health care delivery system and the work force that it employs, but other players (including states, insurers, consumers, and providers) are part of the story as well. Nonetheless, federal policy (both explicit and implicit) has long favored institution-based specialty care and disfavored community-based primary care, and understanding this federal bias is central to the current debate.

Biomedical Research and Institutional Care

The era of American optimism that arrived with the end of World War II brought with it the perception that medical research and specialized medical care would in time conquer nearly all forms of disease. This perception in turn prompted the federal government (through the National Institutes of Health) to funnel billions of dollars to academic medical researchers. And with federal dollars so readily available, medical schools soon emphasized research, and medical students increasingly chose research careers.

Around the same time, Congress enacted the Hill-Burton program, which provided federal funds to stimulate hospital construction and modernization.[9] The policy assumption was that all Americans should have access to the increasingly sophisticated medical care rendered in state-of-the-art hospital facilities. The program gave states federal grants under an allocation system that favored smaller and more rural locations, and the states then dispersed the funds to various hospital projects.[10]

By most accounts, Hill-Burton was an unusually successful federal program: a relatively small fiscal investment (approximately $4 billion) generated nearly 400,000 hospital beds.[11] Many of these were in rural communities. Moreover, the program was popular with state officials (who viewed it as guilt-free pork barrel) and with hospital administrators (who received government funds to build expensive facilities and then received generous insurance reimbursement to deliver hospital care).[12] Not surprisingly, the nation eventually developed an oversupply of hospital beds (which continues today), and Congress finally defunded the program in the late 1970s.[13] Nonetheless, Hill-Burton, along with research funded by the National Institutes of Health, established and promoted the federal bias toward specialized institutional care that still exists.

Expanding the Physician Supply

Hill-Burton and the National Institutes of Health each had an indirect effect on the medical work force, but federal policies beginning in the 1960s had a more direct and important effect. Following a series of reports suggesting a nationwide shortage of physicians,[14] Congress enacted programs designed to increase the overall supply of physicians, encourage the new recruits to become generalists, and encourage more generalists to practice in poor and rural communities.

The first item on the agenda was to increase overall medical school enrollments significantly. Congress awarded federal funding to those medical schools that increased their enrollments. Schools that surpassed their enrollment targets received bonus grants. And medical students received low-interest federal loans.[15] These federal policies, together with the growing popularity and prestige associated with a career in medicine, fueled a remarkable increase in the number of entering medical students. In 1961, for example, there were just over 8,000 first-year medical students; by the mid-1980s, the number was up to around 16,000 (where it remains today).[16]

Congress also encouraged increases in the number of foreign-trained physicians. In 1965, for example, Congress amended the Immigration and Nationality Act to grant preferential immigration status to foreign-born physicians. Over the next decade, thousands of physician immigrants entered the country, many working in poor rural areas and many others working as house staff for urban safety net hospitals.[17] To be sure, the number of physician immigrants declined during the late 1970s as Congress tightened the admission requirements.[18] Simultaneously, however, the number of physicians born in the United States but trained abroad increased significantly, keeping the total number of foreign-trained physicians quite high. As a result, nearly 22 percent of America's current physician work force is foreign-trained.[19]

With rapidly increasing medical school enrollments and the influx of foreign-trained physicians, the overall physician supply rose dramatically. In 1970, for example, the nation had approximately 327,000 physicians, or about 157 physicians for every 100,000 citizens; by 1991, there were over 620,000 physicians, or about 244 for every 100,000 citizens.[20]

As the physician work force expanded, however, it became clear that most of the new recruits were entering specialist careers. In 1940, for example, 64 percent of the nation's physicians were generalists; by 1970 the figure was below 30 percent.[21] There are numerous reasons for this pattern. Specialists' income is generally higher than that received by generalists. Specialists also have higher status and prestige, particularly within the health profession community. Medical schools clearly encourage students to specialize: schools recruit and admit students with strong backgrounds in science (who are often interested in medical research); medical school curricula emphasize the specialties (and generally deemphasize primary care); and medical school faculty (who become student role models) are themselves usually specialists. In addition, when students graduate from medical school and begin their medical residencies, they encounter teaching hospitals that also encourage specialist residencies: not only do specialist residents provide faculty with time to pursue their own research, but such residents generate much more income for hospitals than do generalist residents.

Without doubt, federal policy has encouraged and promoted the emphasis on specialization. Not only did the federal policies just discussed encourage dramatic increases in the physician work force, but (as discussed below) the federal medicare program pays much of the bill for specialist training. But the trend toward specialization has long prompted concern about a shortage of generalists; therefore, beginning in the mid-1960s, federal programs were enacted to encourage generalist practitioners. In the late 1960s and early 1970s, for example, Congress provided federal grants both for generalist health profession students and for medical schools with family practice programs.[22] Congress also declared in 1976 that unless 50 percent of all first-year residents were in generalist residencies by 1980, it would allow only those schools that met the target to receive these grants (an initiative not dissimilar to the residency mandate proposed now by President Clinton).[23]

By and large, however, the efforts to increase the percentage of generalist physicians did not succeed. The share of all physicians who are generalists remains at approximately one-third, and less than 20 percent of first-year residents choose generalist practices.[24] The shortcomings of the generalist initiatives were due to four factors. First, the federal fiscal commitment to these efforts was, from the beginning, rather minimal. Second, funding for the programs was cut even further during the early 1980s, shortly after Ronald Reagan became president. Third, the Graduate Medical Education National Advisory Committee declared in 1981 that the nation would soon have an overall physician surplus. And last, the minimal generalist initiatives never altered the culture of specialization, particularly since other federal programs, such as medicare, continued to nurture that culture.

Throughout the 1960s, the trend toward specialization only exacerbated the geographic maldistribution of doctors. More and more doctors practiced lucrative specialties in affluent communities; fewer and fewer offered primary care to poor and rural communities. In response to this problem, Congress created the National Health Service Corps (NHSC).[25] Under this program, the federal government provides tuition assistance to medical students and other health care professionals who agree to work for at least two years in a medically underserved community.

Although the NHSC scholarship program was always small (at its height, in 1980, the NHSC received approximately $80 million in federal dollars), the effort was relatively successful. By the late 1980s, for example, the program had awarded approximately 22,000 scholarships (mostly to doctors). The program was especially valuable to the nation's federally funded community health clinics: in 1989, for example, NHSC doctors constituted about half of the clinics' physician work force. Moreover, the number of physicians needed to eliminate the nation's health professions shortage areas began to decline (from 4,525 in 1984 to 4,104 in 1988).[26]

By the early 1980s, however, Reagan administration officials were trying to eliminate the NHSC, arguing that it was neither necessary nor desirable. In the words of a high-ranking Reagan appointee, "competition will sort out the major issues of distribution, specialty choice, and workforce mix."[27] As a result, by 1985 the program was largely defunded: thirty-four physicians received NHSC scholarships in that year, compared with over 2,500 awards in 1978.[28]

To be sure, NHSC supporters continued to push the program, and the political environment eventually became more receptive. In 1991, for example, 287 physicians received awards.[29] Moreover, Congress has enacted some incremental efforts to encourage more primary care practitioners for medically underserved communities (the Disadvantaged Minority Health Improvement Act of 1990 and the Health Professions Education Extension Amendments of 1992 are two examples). But the funding levels for these programs are utterly inadequate, and the nation has not yet recovered from the dismantling of the NHSC. For example, the number of physicians needed to eliminate health professions shortage areas is now rising. Moreover, the federally funded community health clinics now have nearly 800 unfilled physician positions, out of a projected physician work force of under 3,000. And almost 43 million Americans now live in health professions shortage areas (indeed, in some communities there is only one physician for every 15,000 residents).[30]

Medicaid and Medicare

The federal bias toward institutional care is also apparent in the reimbursement provisions of the medicaid and medicare programs. Under the medicaid program, enacted by Congress in 1965, the federal government contributes to the cost of state-administered health insurance programs for the poor so long as the state programs comply with a range of federal rules and regulations. The federal rules governing provider reimbursement have limited state flexibility in setting hospital reimbursement rates (and ensured that such rates stay at relatively high levels) while granting states nearly unfettered discretion in setting the rates for office-based physician visits (allowing states to pay doctors at extraordinarily low rates).

The story begins in 1966, with the federal requirement that states reimburse hospitals retrospectively for their actual costs so long as such costs were reasonably related to medicaid patient care. Not surprisingly, this mandate, which followed the reimbursement practices of private insurers, enabled hospitals to recoup nearly all their expenditures, thereby encouraging dramatic increases in hospital spending.

Even the Reagan administration, which in 1981 modified the formula to increase state discretion, still required that hospitals be reimbursed at a "reasonable and adequate rate," a rule that courts often use to require increased reimbursement rates.[31] And while states today have generally abandoned retrospective reimbursement, hospitals remain the best paid of all medicaid providers, receiving payment equal to 82 percent of their actual costs. In contrast, medicaid reimburses outpatient physician care at rates less than half of those provided by private insurance companies. And in some states, such as New York, the medicaid reimbursement for a routine office visit is the absurdly low sum of $11.00.[32]

There is also an obvious bias to medicare's reimbursement system. From 1966 to 1983, medicare (like medicaid) reimbursed hospitals retrospectively for their actual costs. In 1983 Congress enacted the prospective payment system, under which a hospital's reimbursement depends largely on the patient's diagnosis.[33] But Congress also required that teaching hospitals be given a significant bonus to compensate for the higher costs incurred in educating doctors. The direct medical education adjustment reimburses hospitals for a portion of residents' and faculty salaries, and the indirect medical education adjustment reimburses hospitals for the sicker patients and more rigorous care that are generally associated with teaching facilities.

Indeed, Congress was so anxious to protect the teaching facilities that it doubled the indirect adjustment proposed by the federal bureaucrats supervising the program. This fiscal windfall for the teaching hospitals led to a growing reliance on medicare to fund graduate medical education. By 1992, for example, hospitals received $5.2 billion in medicare medical education payments.[34] At no point, however, has Congress used the power of its purse to encourage academic medical centers to increase the number of generalists. To the contrary, Congress has required that medical education payments go only to teaching hospitals, thereby discouraging the growth of ambulatory care training centers, the form of medical education most likely to produce generalist physicians.

Reforming Medical Education: The Current Debate

As discussed above, work force reformers during the 1960s sought to increase the supply of physicians, to encourage physicians to become generalists, and to entice physicians to practice in medically underserved communities. Fifteen years later, the first goal had been accomplished (indeed, a physician surplus was projected by some), and policymakers had generally abandoned the reform agenda. More recently, however, the debate has shifted again, with a consensus emerging on the need for work force reform as a result of several factors. First, it is generally assumed that the rise in health care costs is due, in part, to a surplus of medical specialists.[35] Second, by the early 1990s the number of graduating medical students choosing generalist residencies had reached all-time lows.[36] Third, the growth of the managed-care industry has generated increased demand for generalists (most health maintenance organizations seek a generalist-specialist ratio of 50-50), but market forces have yet to produce the needed supply.[37] And fourth, reform advocates argue convincingly that the geographical maldistribution of the physician work force has worsened significantly during the 1980s.

By 1993 several respected health policy organizations had proposed a similar reform agenda: cap the number of medical residents; create a national physician work force commission to allocate residency slots and require that at least 50 percent be in generalist specialties; provide medicare funding for medical education to ambulatory care facilities; and reduce the maldistribution of the physician work force (through a variety of ill-defined incentive programs).[38] Senator Jay Rockefeller and Representative Henry Waxman then drew on this consensus when drafting the proposed Primary Care Workforce Act of 1993.[39] The Clinton reform proposal followed similar lines.

With the reform momentum building, even long-time opponents of government planning weighed in with their own less ambitious proposals. The Association of American Medical Colleges, for example, adopted as a goal the proposition that a majority of medical students should be entering generalist fields, though the organization urged that regulatory mandates not be imposed until various voluntary incentive programs had been tried and failed.[40] And even the cautious and conservative American Medical Association acknowledged the need for work force planning and incentive programs to increase the number of generalist physicians.[41]

To be sure, the politics of work force planning poses difficult obstacles for reformers. There is, for example, little political gain in a 55 percent generalist mandate; but the opposition (including medical schools and teaching hospitals) is organized and influential. Similarly, the budget deficit makes unlikely any significant federal effort to recruit health professionals to poor and rural communities, particularly since, here again, the constituency favoring such spending is weak and dispersed.

There is also an ongoing debate over the need to have a majority of graduating medical students entering generalist fields. Although the percentage of generalist physicians has declined precipitously since 1960, the actual ratio of generalists to population during that same period has remained relatively constant (at approximately 75 generalists per 100,000 population).[42] The problem, however, is that there was a dramatic decline in the percentage of medical students choosing generalist careers in the 1980s, thus suggesting a shortage of generalists in years to come (particularly with the recent emphasis on managed-care organizations). In 1982, for example, 36.1 percent of graduating medical students entered generalist specialties (42.7 percent including obstetrics and gynecology); by 1992 the figure was down to 14.6 percent (17.3 percent including obstetrics and gynecology).[43] In Texas, for example, 42 percent of the state's rural family practice physicians will retire in the next five years, and the medical training pipeline has few trainees preparing to replace them.[44]

However, it may be possible to avoid a shortage of generalists if even 30 percent of graduating medical students choose generalist careers and if the nation produces more nonphysician providers, such as nurse-practitioners and physician assistants.[45] Moreover, as managed-care organizations compete for generalists, thereby increasing generalists' income, the market itself may resolve the problem. Indeed, this may be starting already. In 1993, for the first time in a decade, the percentage of first-year residents choosing generalist specialties rose, to 19.3 percent (or 22.4 percent including obstetrics and gynecology).[46]

Despite the political pitfalls and the uncertainty over numbers, a Congress anxious to enact bold health care reform—but wary of employer mandates, premium caps, and regional health alliances—just might pass the 55 percent mandate into law. After all, such an initiative promises simultaneously to revolutionize the medical work force, improve the quality of medical care, and save money. Moreover, although a major effort to reduce the maldistribution of physicians is unlikely, some incremental programs along this line seem inevitable.

Work Force Reform: Obstacles and Opportunities

It is important to consider carefully the implementation obstacles work force reform is likely to encounter. By doing so now, before the enactment of a new law, Congress could (and should) enact a more feasible and functional reform agenda.

Regulating Residencies

Any attempt to mandate residency allotments has an Achilles' heel: the lengthy medical training pipeline. Assume, for example, that Congress immediately enacted the 55 percent mandate, adopting as national policy the proposition that the nation needs a 50-50 generalist-specialist ratio. Assume also that such a mandate was implemented without a hitch (hardly a realistic assumption). Rather remarkably, even under this all too rosy scenario, the 50-50 ratio would not be reached until the year 2040.[47] Moreover, given the implementation obstacles likely to occur, the 50-50 ratio may just be unattainable (which may not be all bad).

Legislation that caps the overall number of medical residents and requires that 55 percent of all entering residents be generalists by 1998 would have an enormous impact on medical schools, teaching hospitals (and safety net hospitals more generally), medical students, nonphysician providers, the middle class, the states, and the federal government.

MEDICAL SCHOOLS. In 1992 eighteen medical schools received grants from the Robert Wood Johnson Foundation to plan programs to generate interest in generalist careers. More than two-thirds of the nation's medical schools had applied for these grants.[48] In mid-1994, up to twelve of the eighteen received six-year implementation grants of $2.5 million each. The initiative, still in its infancy, already suggests two lessons: first, most medical schools will pursue incremental generalist agendas (particularly if someone else foots the bill); and second, changing the medical school educational environment is a difficult and daunting task that requires planning, funding, and phasing.

Indeed, as any student of bureaucracy knows, implementing the fundamental restructuring of an established institution is never easy. This is especially true of medical schools, given the numerous institutional changes required, the culture and character of the organizations themselves, and the fifty-year history of federal encouragement of specialty-based training. For example, a generalist agenda requires medical schools to alter their admissions criteria (to seek a more diverse student body), curricula (to emphasize the importance of a generalist career), faculty composition (both to teach the new curricula and to provide generalist role models), rotation requirements (to create links with ambulatory care sites), and research priorities (to acknowledge the importance of primary care research).

Moreover, this organizational revolution is to be designed and implemented by the specialists and subspecialists who now dominate the institutions, who have themselves promoted and profited from the trend toward specialization, and who are both influential and organized. (The former director of the Mississippi Health Department suggests that the dean of the Mississippi Medical School had more political influence than he did.)[49]

Nor is medical school resistance explainable solely by organizational politics. Medical schools could suffer significant fiscal losses as they shift to a generalist emphasis. Indeed, medical schools now receive one-third of their income from third-party reimbursement received by faculty practice plans (most of which is generated by specialists).[50]

TEACHING HOSPITALS. Like the medical schools, teaching hospitals oppose caps and mandates: residents are an inexpensive source of physician labor, they generate significant revenue, and they enable teaching faculty to engage in important and ongoing research. Teaching hospitals are also worried about the residency allocation process, under which the national council on graduate medical education would assign slots based not only on historical distribution but on the quality of individual facilities, the need for racial and ethnic diversity, and the recommendations of physicians and consumers.[51] Implementing these allocation criteria among almost 7,000 training programs around the country will be difficult, subjective, and political. Teaching hospitals in some states, such as New York, are especially worried about how they will fare under a political allocation process.[52]

More generally, teaching hospitals (like medical safety net institutions more generally) worry about their economic viability in a world of managed competition. These are high-cost institutions: it is expensive to train doctors, conduct research, and treat rare diseases.[53] To be sure, the Health Security Act acknowledges this problem, both with the requirement that health plans contract with academic medical centers to treat patients with rare diseases and with the creation of an all-payer pool to provide teaching facilities with a $9.6 billion supplemental payment by the year 2000.[54] But the hospitals insist that the proposed subsidy is inadequate (indeed less than they would get without reform under current funding streams). This issue is especially important since institutions struggling to survive will have trouble successfully implementing the organizational revolution required to produce more generalists.

The proposed cap on the total number of first-year medical residents also has implications for the medical safety net. Although the Clinton plan leaves to federal bureaucrats the task of setting that cap, many analysts propose figures between 105 percent and 115 percent of the nation's graduating medical class. (By way of contrast, the number today is around 135 percent. This number includes graduates of American medical schools, foreign-trained students, and students who took time off between medical school and residency programs.) The goal, clearly, is to reduce the number of foreign-trained residents (who now make up approximately 25 percent of first-year residents).[55] But foreign-trained residents serve poor and rural communities in disproportionate numbers, and the reductions proposed could well harm the ability of safety net institutions to care for the needy. It would indeed be ironic if national work force reform resulted in fewer doctors for the poor.

MEDICAL STUDENTS. According to a former medical school administrator, if he were a program director, he would have "no idea how to convince—or coerce—half of the graduating residents to pursue careers as generalists."[56] To be sure, in a world of mandates students would not need to be convinced. Instead, those who applied unsuccessfully for a specialist placement would have no choice but to accept a generalist position. (How this process would work is unclear: would there be a "generalist default" category during the national residency matching program?) But the generalists produced by such a regulatory regime may not be the generalists the nation needs: reluctant generalists may not be very good ones, and they are particularly unlikely to practice in medically underserved communities, which is where generalists are most needed.

The better solution, of course, is to recruit and admit medical students who are interested in generalist careers and to provide a curriculum and a faculty that nurture that interest. But achieving such fundamental change would be a slow process, and in the meantime student resistance is a likely implementation obstacle.

NONPHYSICIAN PROVIDERS. The medical work force debate is complicated significantly by the presence of nonphysician providers (particularly nurse-practitioners, nurse midwives, and physician assistants), most of whom provide good, relatively low-cost primary care to an otherwise underserved population. For example, more than 80 percent of the nation's 30,000 nurse-practitioners work in primary care settings, and over half work with the medically underserved. Similarly, approximately half of the nation's 23,500 physician assistants work in primary care practices, many in rural communities.[57] As a result, many health care analysts call for an increased supply of these providers.[58] Interestingly, however, there are two somewhat inconsistent rationales offered in support of an expansionist policy. First, given the long physician training pipeline, nonphysician providers, who can be trained quickly and cheaply, can help fill the generalist gap.[59] But a short-term reliance on nonphysician providers threatens their utility once the generalist physician pipeline is producing results: at that point there may be an oversupply of generalists.

Second, studies suggest and advocates argue that nonphysician providers can provide medical services within their expertise just as well as physicians.[60] Since most nonphysician providers work as generalists, the need for generalist physicians decreases as the number of nonphysician providers increases. This of course suggests again that a 50-50 generalist-specialist physician ratio may not be necessary (and may lead to an oversupply of generalists).

Unfortunately, however, the effort to produce more nonphysician providers is complicated and difficult. First, federal funding to train nonphysician providers was cut significantly during the 1980s. Physician assistant programs, for example, now receive only 62 percent of the federal funds provided in 1981.[61]

Second, there is ongoing intramural battling among the various health policy communities: doctors are reluctant to cede authority to nurses, and doctors and nurses both are wary of physician assistants. As one doctor put it, allowing nurse-practitioners additional independence "will send the message loud and clear to the medical students: 'Why bother to go into family care? You can go to nurse practitioner school.' I spent 11 years in medical school, and you're telling me someone else could do it better and for less money with less education? That's ludicrous."[62] These turf battles are generally dominated by organized medicine, leading to various "scope of practice" laws (which limit activities of nonphysician providers) and to insurer reluctance to reimburse care by nonphysician providers.

And third, efforts to alter these patterns and practices face strong and organized resistance. For example, Texas has made efforts to increase significantly the supply of nonphysician providers. However, according to the director of the Texas medicaid program, "that is very hard to do . . . through the legislative process, because of the politics of medicine and their power to stop it. In fact, we had difficulty just getting nurse practitioners to be able to be [medicaid] reimbursed. . . . [Doctors] didn't want to let the nurses get in under the tent."[63]

To be sure, the Clinton plan calls for the override of inappropriate laws regulating the scope of practice. The Health Security Act states that "no state may, through licensure or otherwise, restrict the practice of any class of health professionals beyond what is justified by the skills and training of such professionals."[64] But the provision is far too vague, and it simply adds the federal government to the parties involved in litigation that challenges laws restricting the scope of practice.

THE MIDDLE CLASS. Often lost in the debate over work force policy is the fact that most Americans, at least those with private insurance or medicare coverage, already have a physician whom they see on a regular basis (a "principal physician"). Moreover, these principal physicians are not always generalists: one study suggests that 20 percent of the population receives their principal care from a specialist.[65] And for many Americans, ready access to the best available specialty care is the most positive feature of the entire health care system (thus the ongoing resistance to those health maintenance organizations that significantly limit freedom of choice).

The middle class, in other words, is generally happy with the medical work force available to it, which suggests caution about the political wisdom of efforts to revise the work force composition. To be sure, the long medical training pipeline means that any reduction in specialists will not be felt for years to come. Nonetheless, the adverse political reaction to a residency mandate could well be significant, and public opinion could easily become another important implementation obstacle.[66]

THE STATES. States are key players in America's health care system.[67] Moreover, the Clinton plan delegates to the states numerous new tasks, including the responsibility for ensuring that all citizens have access to a choice of high-quality health plans.[68] But while states must (theoretically, anyway) guarantee that the work force in all communities is adequate, it is federal officials (in the proposed national council on graduate medical education) who would shape the actual work force by capping the number of first-year medical residents, allocating residencies by specialty, ensuring that 55 percent were in primary care, and assigning residency positions to specific programs.

The decision to nationalize the efforts to produce more generalists would significantly affect state-based activities to control the supply of health care providers. During the late 1980s, for example, nearly every state implemented new programs to recruit more generalists and to persuade the new recruits to practice in medically underserved communities. These state initiatives were prompted, in large part, by the dramatic reduction in federal efforts to increase the number of generalist providers.[69] Since many of the state efforts are only recently under way, it is too soon to tell whether they are working. It is clear, however, that under the Clinton plan, the federal government would assume responsibility for the task of producing more generalists, while the states would retain primary responsibility for solving the problem of geographic maldistribution.

Not all state officials oppose an increased federal role. It is generally acknowledged, for example, that state-based regulation of medical education is often too fragmented, with authority divided between state education departments and state health departments. This decentralization of authority, combined with the significant influence commanded by academic medical centers, makes it difficult for state health officials to enact substantive work force reform. As a Texas official notes, "as long as decisionmaking is left to the state level to try to come up with the incentives and requirements. . . . I am not very confident that we are going to catch up anytime soon."[70]

Moreover, 56.2 percent of the nation's medical residents are trained in only eight states (15 percent in New York State alone).[71] This uneven distribution also suggests that residency allocation, if done at all, should be done nationally: why should New York allocate residency slots for doctors who are trained in New York but will practice elsewhere?

But if national decisionmaking is justified in principle, state officials are nervous about the implementation. For example, because of the interstate variation in training programs, any allocation system that emphasizes generalists and distributes dollars and doctors to a subset of 7,500 training programs around the country is sure to downsize the resident population in New York. Indeed, New York expects a 20 percent reduction in first-year slots.[72] Conversely, as other states seek more from the allocation process and are supported in that quest by their congressional delegations, the possibility that the entire process could degenerate into pork barrel politics looms large.

Making the allocation process even more complicated, however, are two facts: nearly two-thirds of the nation's medical schools are state schools, and most public hospitals are teaching hospitals. Since state education officials surely will resist ceding authority to federal health regulators, and since municipal hospital administrators will be similarly disinclined, there is sure to be significant intergovernmental tension (and litigation).

THE FEDERAL GOVERNMENT. There is, finally, the question of federal capacity: the effort to regulate and allocate medical residencies requires staff and skills well beyond what now exists. To be sure, there are public officials well versed in work force issues. Staffers in the Bureau of Health Professions (a relatively small unit within the Department of Health and Human Services) have long worked on provider supply issues. Similarly, the Council on Graduate Medical Education, created by Congress in 1986, has as its mission the review and analysis of work force trends, and the Physician Payment Review Commission also has staff assigned to this topic.

But even if the new national council on graduate medical education and the new national institute for health care work force development recruit heavily from these various agencies (or from similar agencies now in place in state governments), the tasks assigned and skills required go well beyond anything now in place. For example, staff is needed to determine (annually) an appropriate number of first-year residents, to determine how many residencies should be in each specialty (hardly a precise science), to rank the 7,500 teaching programs (according to quality criteria not yet developed), to factor in the need for diversity, and to negotiate the political minefield that will inevitably accompany the actual allotment of positions.[73] These are all difficult tasks, especially when one considers the interest groups vying to shape the process.

This is not to suggest, of course, that the proposed new agency, if established, will not over time hire capable and committed staff. Nor is it to suggest that staffing this agency would be more difficult than staffing other institutions proposed in the Clinton plan (such as regional health alliances). It does suggest, however, that the tasks assigned to the new workers may be particularly difficult for federal bureaucrats to implement. Indeed, even the current Council on Graduate Medical Education, one of the strongest and most effective advocates for a generalist mandate, opposes federal efforts to allocate residency slots. According to the council, there should be community-based private-sector consortia, composed of medical schools, teaching hospitals, consumers, and others, that should be assigned this task. As a council representative argued recently before Congress:

> The consortium proposal does not attempt to define at the national level the exact number of residency positions that should be offered in each of the 81 specialties at each institution. COGME believes that this task would be extraordinarily difficult, would provide excessive micromanagement of the system, and should be accomplished at the local level.[74]

Implementation Analysis and Agenda Setting

All too often, policymakers enact new policies without thinking through the hard questions of implementation: what institutions will perform what tasks; are such tasks feasible; and what problems are likely to emerge? Indeed, rather than confronting such issues, federal policymakers often establish broad (and perhaps unreachable) goals and delegate to others (federal bureaucrats, state officials, private contractors) the task of implementation. All too often, the result is a program beset by problems and academic studies suggesting that government is inept and inadequate.

Admittedly, even the best-planned government programs inevitably encounter implementation problems. To suggest otherwise is naive. But in this chapter I have discussed why the implementation of a mandate requiring 55 percent of all new residents to be generalists would be especially difficult. First, there are fifty years of federal policy encouraging specialty-based institutional care. Second, the institutional revolution required to institute the mandate (in medical schools, teaching hospitals, and elsewhere) will be hard to achieve. And third, even if the institutional change were easy to accomplish, the medical training pipeline is so long that producing a 50-50 generalist-specialist ratio would still take almost fifty years.

There are times, of course, when implementation obstacles are no excuse for rejecting legislation. An obvious example is civil rights legislation: southern resistance to integration made implementing the policy both more difficult and more important. Nonetheless, the medical work force issues discussed here are far more ambiguous. First, there is the underlying uncertainty about the need for 55 percent of first-year residents to be generalists. There is reason to believe, for example, that if 30 percent of the first-year students are generalists and if the nation promotes the training of nonphysician providers, the overall medical work force will be close to where it should be.

Second, and even more important, the national effort to cap and regulate residencies diverts attention from a more serious (and more manageable) problem: the shortage of providers of all types in poor and rural communities. The need now is for a national effort to remedy the problem of maldistribution: mandates and caps that govern the overall supply and mix of the physician population can and should wait for another day. This is especially true since the overall reform effort may have the ironic and unintended effect of reducing the work force available to the poor, both by reducing the number of residents available in urban teaching hospitals and by threatening the viability of many safety net institutions.

To be sure, the Clinton plan contains various proposals to address the maldistribution problem, such as increased funding for the National Health Service Corps. The goal is that by the year 2005 there will be 8,000 corps practitioners (up from the current 1,600).[75] There are also tax incentives provided to health professionals who work in underserved communities, and there is federal funding for new community health clinics.

But these efforts should be expanded significantly, particularly since programs like the National Health Service Corps seem to work, when given a chance. There should be, for example, a commitment to expanding the corps well beyond the administration's incremental (though not insignificant) proposals. Also needed are a well-funded program to forgive student loans in return for work in medically underserved communities; increased reimbursement to physicians who work in underserved communities; and significant expansion of programs like the Federal Health Careers Opportunities Program, which encourages and enables minority youngsters to pursue careers in the health professions. There should also be a major effort to expand the number of federally funded community health clinics. In other words, there should be a national commitment to reducing the maldistribution of the medical work force.

Indeed, in many ways the Clinton work force proposals conflict with two basic principles suggested by implementation analysis. The first principle is that a program that is unusually difficult to implement (such as the 55 percent mandate) should be implemented only if it is a measured response to an important problem (not the case here). The second principle is that a program that successfully addresses an ongoing problem (such as the National Health Service Corps) should be emphasized and expanded.

This is not to suggest, however, that the effort to recast federal policy away from encouraging institution-based specialty care and toward community-based generalist care is misguided. Nor am I suggesting that Congress should not use the power of its purse to increase the number of first-year generalist residents. The need for congressional action was particularly clear when less than 15 percent of first-year residents were choosing generalist residencies, and although the number is now higher (around 20 percent), it should be higher still (30 percent may be enough). Congress should, for example, provide medical schools with fiscal incentives to increase their emphasis on generalist programs. (It could even help fund programs like the Robert Wood Johnson Generalist Physician Initiative.) Congress also should change the medicare rules for graduate medical education to encourage ambulatory site facilities (or even community-based consortia) to receive federal funds to train medical residents (although such a shift would, of course, reduce teaching hospital revenues).

But the Clinton work force proposals should be directed away from an emphasis on specialty maldistribution and toward solving the problem of geographic maldistribution. Not only is geographic maldistribution the more pressing problem, it also is a policy arena in which there are tried and tested government programs (such as the National Health Service Corps and the community health clinics). Specialty maldistribution, in contrast, presents a more complex and uncertain policy arena, in which both the nature of the problem and the certainty of the solution are less clear. In this context, the rapid imposition of an overall cap on the number of medical residents and a 55 percent mandate hardly seems warranted, although I should emphasize again that an incremental response need not be inconsequential.

Despite these criticisms, President Clinton and his staff are surely correct when they argue that the United States needs a new medical work force policy. Moreover, the plan as presented, along with the debate over health care reform, provides a window for strong federal action. Congress and the president should work together to develop a revised work force policy that emphasizes the need to reduce the geographic maldistribution of health professionals. By doing so, the federal government would go a long way toward solving the health care crisis.

6 ||| An Ounce of Implementation Needs a Pound of Policy Foresight

John J. DiIulio, Jr., Donald F. Kettl, and
Gerald Garvey

THE CHAPTERS in this volume have discussed the specific administrative opportunities and challenges of reforming the nation's health care complex. Together, the chapters provide scores of ideas and recommendations for ways to make health care reform work. But each warns that an ounce of foresight about how to carry out policy can be worth a pound of poorly administered or unimplemented policy cures. Consider just five examples.

—*Welfare reform: policy déjà vu.* In 1988 a Democratic Congress passed, and a Republican president signed, the Family Support Act. Title II of the act, the Job Opportunities and Basic Skills (JOBS) program, was designed to change fundamentally the way the states administered certain public assistance programs by emphasizing so-called workfare. Six years later, in most states nothing much had happened. The implementation problems with the Family Support Act were many but fixable. Federal policymakers, however, ignored the problems; in 1994 they began to debate a new workfare-oriented reform plan that, if enacted, would broaden the reach of the as yet unimplemented 1988 law.[1]

—*Environmental protection: toxic implementation.* In 1970 a presidential reorganization created the Environmental Protection Agency. In the past quarter century the EPA has been the principal agency charged with carrying out legislation on air and water pollution and toxic waste cleanup. The agency's effectiveness has been limited, however, by various administrative problems, some of its own making but most imposed on it by the very lawmakers of both parties who insist that it do a better job. In creating the Superfund program, for example, Congress set a ceiling on the share of the program's funds that could be spent on staff. As a result, the EPA was forced to delegate most Superfund operations and many policy decisions to private contractors. The EPA lacked the managerial capacity to oversee this network of contractors, and Superfund's slim staff was plagued by high rates of turnover.[2] The unsurprising result: scandals, cost overruns, and precious few toxic waste sites cleaned up.

—*Youth and families: inconsistent programs.* In the 1980s some thirty states, aided by the federal government, embarked on experiments with so-called family preservation programs intended to keep troubled families together and children out of foster care. Most of the programs involved intensive family counseling and social services. But in 1993 the largest and most rigorous study of the programs concluded that they did nothing to keep families together or reduce child neglect or abuse.[3]

It would have been a miracle, however, if the programs had worked. State child welfare systems are plagued by excessive caseloads, sloppy record-keeping, poor training, and other basic administrative problems. Most state and local agencies responsible for abused, neglected, and delinquent children living at home, with foster families, or in group homes and facilities are cesspools of bureaucratic mismanagement and waste. Meanwhile, the federal government adds national confusion to subnational turmoil by loosely administering numerous separate programs for youth and families.[4]

Even such a highly touted federal program as Head Start is rife with administrative problems. Head Start comprises 2,000 separate programs operating in 36,000 classrooms. There are no standard personnel selection processes, wide differences in the enforcement of policies governing parental involvement, and so on.[5] Research has failed to show that Head Start has any lasting effects on IQ, the incidence of teen pregnancy and employment, or the growth of welfare dependency and crime.[6] But no one can say for sure whether Head Start works because what Head Start is varies so much from one setting to the next.

—*Crime: federalism and responsibility.* In 1993 the U.S. Senate approved a $22 billion package of anticrime legislation. The bill included $8.9 billion for 100,000 additional local police. Almost no thought, however, was given to how this massive new intergovernmental program might be implemented or how its effects might be measured and evaluated. For example, the bill provided that within six years after localities had received the money they would have to find the funds to keep the new cops on the beat. These community policing provisions were to be administered by the Bureau of Justice Assistance, an agency that has experienced great difficulties in keeping its annual $400 million block grant program from running amok.[7]

The BJA is the chief administrative successor to the Law Enforcement Assistance Administration, which was established by the 1968 Omnibus Crime Control and Safe Streets Act. In fiscal year 1972 the LEAA's budget was larger than the total budget for the Justice Department in fiscal year 1968. By 1980 the agency had spent billions on state and local anticrime efforts, including seed money for community-oriented policing initiatives. But the LEAA was regarded as a terrible failure.[8] From its inception it was plagued by administrative problems that neither its early boosters nor its later critics ever seemed to acknowledge. The agency and its dozens of programs were not designed with the realities of intergovernmental relations in mind. The LEAA passed out the federal dollars, but it did not shape the policy or modify the administration of subnational criminal justice agencies.

—*Transportation: conflicting requirements*. In 1956 Congress passed the Federal Aid Highway Act. In 28 pages, it "authorized the interstate highway system, levied the taxes to pay for it, and established the trust fund that would receive the tax receipts and disburse them for construction projects." The highways got built. In 1991 Congress passed the Intermodal Surface Transportation Efficiency Act. The law ran to 293 pages. In addition to finishing the highways and aiding mass transit, it mandated that the responsible bureaucrats in Washington and the states "relieve [traffic] congestion, improve air quality, preserve historic sites, encourage the use of auto seat belts and motorcycle helmets, control erosion and storm water runoff, monitor traffic and collect data on speeding, reduce drunk driving . . . use recycled paper in making asphalt . . . control the use of calcium magnesium acetate in performing seismic retrofits on bridges," and much, much more.[9]

What the law did not specify was how the Department of Transportation, the Federal Highway Administration, the Urban Mass Transit Administration, or the fifty state transportation agencies were to achieve these competing objectives or manage the inevitable trade-offs among them. Nevertheless, within two years federal policymakers began to ask why the money Congress had appropriated was "being spent so slowly, and why the transit systems it authorized were so long in taking shape."[10]

It would be a relief if these examples were exceptions to the rule. Unfortunately, they are anything but. In the past few years the failure of public management inside the beltway has meant medicare fraud, the flawed Hubble Space Telescope, some of the worst defense procurement scandals ever, skyrocketing defaults in the guaranteed student loan program, and malfeasance of Teapot Dome proportions in the Department of Housing and Urban Development.[11]

There is no shortage of scholarship, which began to appear in the 1970s, analyzing failures of policy implementation and public service reform. In 1972, for example, Martha Derthick reported on a federal program intended to make federal surplus lands available to cities for the development of low-income housing. Her main finding: except for two sites (at which only 300 housing units were constructed), the projects were never begun.[12] And in 1973 Jeffrey Pressman and Aaron Wildavsky reported on a small federal program intended to bring jobs to Oakland, California. Their chief finding: only a few hundred jobs of 3,000 promised were ever created.[13] In both cases, and in scores more since, implementation of promising policies was scuttled by failure to plan, failure to follow through, and failure to have the patience to work out the bugs.

A Cautionary Administrative Analogy

Health reform need not furnish material for the next generation of studies on failed implementation. If policymakers acknowledge the basic realities of federalizing, implementing, and managing health care reform summarized in chapter 1, reform can work. But no one should expect it to work flawlessly or with great speed. Perhaps the single most instructive administrative analogy is to the quarter-century-old attempt to reform the nation's environmental protection system.

Between 1970 and 2000 the United States will have constructed the most comprehensive and complicated body of environmental laws, regulations, and policies in the world. For the most part, Congress and federal regulators have taken the lead. The states and many cities have followed suit, frequently to the extent of passing laws and rules more stringent than minimum national standards.

A handful of federal statutes frame the U.S. environmental regime.

These include, most notably, the National Environmental Protection Act (NEPA), the Clean Air Act (CAA), the Clean Water Act, the Toxic Substances Control Act (TOSCA), and the Resource Conservation and Recovery Act (RCRA). In total pages of the U.S. Code, these statutes together substantially exceed the number represented by the Clinton administration's draft Health Security Act. The working portions of the environmental framework, however, probably give a useful point of reference because they arguably suggest the magnitude and complexity of the president's proposed health care regime.

The early works of federal environmental legislation turned out to be an invitation to a complex, continuing process that has taken innumerable turns not foreseen by the planners of the first Earth Day. One must expect federal health care reform legislation to follow a similar evolutionary course.

Significant in this connection is the overall time needed for implementation. The basic structure of the environmental regime will have taken three decades to construct (taking passage of NEPA and the first major version of the CAA, both in 1970, as the starting point and completion of a national emissions trading system for acid rain credits in 2000 as the completion point). But the Clinton administration's Health Security Act plan, or any plan similar to it in scope and timetable, would call for the installation, in not more than a half-dozen years from the time of passage, of a national health care regime that is of at least the magnitude of an environmental regime that—a quarter century after Americans got serious about ecology—is still in the process of becoming.

The experience with the environmental regime is instructive in additional ways. Soon after the passage of the early versions of the clean air and clean water legislation, it became evident that complex issues with regional variations could not be satisfactorily dealt with by congressional fiat. Gradually, a series of statutory adjustments were made and state and local regulatory institutions and procedures emerged to implement the cleanup policy. For air pollution cleanup and control, for example, federal law directly relates to most mobile sources of airborne pollutants and to major new (at the time of the laws' passage) stationary sources. State governments remain responsible for policies and implementation applicable to preexisting stationary sources—most of the nation's factories and electric generating plants. Surpassingly elaborate SIPs (state implementation plans) have been worked out, reviewed and approved by the administrator of the Environmental Protection Agency, and frequently revised. Governance in environmental policy is a major industry, not just a handful of programs.

The federal-state-local regime evolved erratically through continuous political negotiation and technical refinement, always with insistent involvement by industry lobbyists and technicians and by representatives of environmental protection groups.

Another point of likely similarity between environmental protection reform and health care reform is in administrative law. The federal statutory framework for environmental matters is enormously detailed, but that fact at no time worked to preclude the need for an even more elaborate body of administrative rules. The federal EPA and its counterpart state and local agencies have probably generated pages of rules and weeks of rulemaking processes for every paragraph of statutory law. And the litigation spawned by environmental legislation, rulemakings, and administrative caselaw has not only inevitably become a growth industry in its own right, but has frequently prevented policies from attaining full settlement until test cases have worked their way through the full appellate hierarchy. Health care reform must be expected to initiate proceedings with similar consequences—lingering uncertainties, horrendous costs, the injection of concepts and considerations external to those of medical or administrative expertise into the policy process.

But the most fundamental parallel is the extent to which health care reform, too, will have to rely on the states to carry out federal policy. This complicates enforcement.

A 1994 General Accounting Office study identified 105 state pollution prevention programs nationwide and found major differences in how they operated. "These programs obtain funding from EPA that rewards their after-the-fact strategies without looking into whether prevention was possible, which is inconsistent with the policy established by the Pollution Prevention Act."[14] Such disjunctures between federal policy and state administrative actions could easily prove just as common in health reform.

Indeed, the word *reform* perhaps implies a well-thought-out, once-and-for-all reconstruction—a recognition that the existing structure is broke but quickly and easily fixable if only decisionmakers approach the task with intelligence, courage, and resolution. Health care procedures in the United States may indeed be broke, and may be fixable, but the analogy of reform of structures to protect the environment suggests that action by Congress will represent only the start of a long process involving enormous bureaucratic growth in Washington and the states, active involvement by the courts, giving-and-taking over a period of decades by relevant interest groups, and future consequences and developments that the framers of today's initiatives cannot even begin to foresee.

Management, Money, and Accountability

One problem they can foresee, however, is the difficulty of institutionalizing accountability for the results of reform. Accountability has always relied on linking management responsibilities with budgetary muscle. From Oriental potentates to modern presidents, decisionmakers have learned that expansive talk about policy is cheap and promises of good management for quick results are easy. Resources can too readily be wasted; only by coupling resources to results can governmental systems be effectively and efficiently managed. Money is the critical resource that makes other resources, from time to skill, possible. Supplying money makes management possible; threatening to remove it always catches the manager's attention. Linking the responsibility for raising and spending money, for taxes and results, has always been the linchpin of accountability.

In health care reform, however, the disconnection between funding and managing makes accountability difficult. Depending on the choice of plans, funds flow into the health care system from private individuals (through payroll deductions), their employers (through mandated contributions), the federal government (through subsidies and payments for medicare and medicaid recipients), and state governments (through cost sharing in the government-funded portion of the program). Funds flow out through a complex network of health care providers, supervised by federal, state, private sector, and nonprofit organizations. Any reform involving purchasing cooperatives or alliances will introduce hybrid organizations. Payers will expect influence over results, but since responsibility for paying will be shared, so too will control over outcomes. Control will be diffused because the outcomes will be shaped by the behavior of networks of different organizations loosely coupled together.

American government, of course, has substantial experience in sharing power in public programs.[15] But the experience has been troubled by confusion over just where authority for decisions rests and by lack of government's capacity to oversee the behavior of its private partners.[16]

Because of its extent, health care reform will magnify the issues and the problems that could result from not solving them.

Solving the problems requires two steps. First, government policymakers must decide where public authority ultimately rests. In a system of shared power created by public officials to pursue public goals, citizens will look to government to solve problems. But on a deeper level, working through this question will require government policymakers to sort out the responsibilities of the participants. Some of these matters are questions of policy design: what role should government assume in assessing and ensuring the quality of health care, for example? Others are questions of process: if a consumer is not happy with the choices offered by competing health plans, or if an interest group believes that an alliance does not serve all citizens equally, lawsuits surely will result.

One further lesson of a quarter century of federal environmental policymaking is that continual legal battles over the distribution of authority and responsibility are inevitable in important programs where public power is shared. Never before in American history have decisionmakers considered a policy of such broad coverage, with literally life and death implications, that has involved such intricate administrative relationships. Any version of health care reform will therefore raise crucial questions of rights and responsibilities, and resolving them will entail substantial litigation and political struggle. And because reform raises tough questions for which neither the administrative nor the legal system now has adequate answers, reform will demand nothing less than a reinvention of the public law covering these issues.

Making health care reform work ultimately depends on building within government the capacity to define and perform its own role. In part this is because of the legal realities of the program: a *public* health care reform program requires defining and exercising public responsibility. And in part, this is because of the administrative realities: exercising public responsibility requires constructing competent centers of public power. In addition, the political realities are that having created health care reform, government officials will be responsible for solving its problems.

The nation could avoid these daunting challenges if it focused on easier problems, but then millions of Americans would be deprived of affordable, quality health care. We could avoid administrative complexity by leaving the program completely in either federal or private hands. We would then have either to accept a truly huge federal bureaucracy or allow some citizens to fall through the cracks of private plans. The fundamental problem of health care reform is that in trying to do hard things, we are seeking to incorporate values of responsiveness and choice along with the goals of efficiency and effectiveness. The search for multiple, complex, and even conflicting goals is the foundation of American federalism. And American federalism—the view from the states—is the inescapable cornerstone of health care reform.

7 || Implementing Health Reform: What the States Face

Lawrence D. Brown

THE UNITED STATES is a society famed for incremental change sustained in part by tests of policy effectiveness in the laboratories of democracy that are the states. Yet as health care reform raced to the top of the national agenda in the early 1990s, the debate quickly narrowed to two alternatives—a single-payer system and managed competition—that no state had ever tried. In addition, the Clinton administration proposed a decidedly nonincremental initiative that would reform the health care delivery system, slow the growth of health care spending to the rate of growth of the consumer price index, and bring secure coverage to all citizens by the end of the decade. If the nation is to achieve affordable universal coverage, whether on the Clinton model and timetable or by more modest measures, the implementation tasks facing state and national policymakers will be enormous. Even if one could predict the final shape of the national health care program—and so far no one can—it would still be impossible to provide detailed responses to these management challenges. Sometimes the past is an instructive prologue, sometimes a disconnected and misleading predictor, and it is hard to judge prospectively when it is the one, the other, or neither. Still, attention to implementation is necessary not so much because it reliably rescues policymakers from an errant course (although occasionally it might do so) but because it can deepen federal and state deliberations about the design of policy and the generic management issues diverse policy designs produce.

Getting Up to Speed

In the United States, affordable universal coverage will surely mean new health care financing arrangements, will probably mean new cost-containment plans, and may perhaps mean significant public efforts to overhaul the delivery system. A new regime will entail more or less constant struggles to balance quality and access against cost in ways that produce value for money. In a sense all Western societies face basically the same health care crisis: high consumer expectations, technological innovation, more demanding concepts of quality, aging populations, and pressures to equalize payments within the expanding medical work force are givens in the health politics of most Western nations. The reason the United States has been slow to grapple effectively with these powerful forces has little to do with their power per se but rather with American distrust of government as an organizing force in society, a distrust unique among Western nations. Other countries have long understood that rational steering of the health care system and defensible balancing of its many conflicting goals require a clear central government policy framework. The United States, by contrast, has clung to a laissez-faire philosophy that leaves the central government interfering in all aspects of the system except the most important ones. In essence, the U.S. health care policy problem is a government problem or, better put, a problem the United States has with the role of government. Affordable universal coverage cannot work without a firm end to laissez-faire, without the federal government's assumption of new directive responsibilities and powers that would create an entitlement, define basic benefits, establish a stable financing system, reform health insurance practices, and promote cost containment.

Although new federal leadership is crucial to any coherent reform package, how, and how well, a new health care system works will depend importantly on how, and how well, the states put it in place. The Canadian single-payer system is made up of ten provincial systems linked by a succinct but serviceable set of national rules. The Clinton version of managed competition relies heavily on state implementation, and so too, probably, will any program with enough political support to become law.

The states' duties are unlikely to wither away under national health care reform for several reasons. First, the specter of "excessive" federal control could doom the passage of a bill, which encourages devolving various duties onto subnational governments. Second, the states have started (and in a few cases even moved) down the road to reforms of their own and will resist scrapping them merely because the federal government belatedly has its own notion. In addition, states have long regulated insurance companies, licensed health care providers, promoted public health, reviewed capital expenditures, and performed other functions that few reformers would propose entirely to federalize. States have health care economies with substantially varying wages, prices, resources, and popular preferences, so no detailed national blueprint for the rationalization of the "industry" will be acceptable. And, not least important, political bargaining in Washington over divisive legislative issues will probably trigger a time-honored coalition-building strategy—pass into law a combination of vaguely worded statutory language and constraining legislative details and delegate the caboodle to the states with fine print warning that some assembly is required.

The impressive legacy of state prerogatives in overseeing health care might seem to imply that affordable universal coverage is but the next logical step in an incrementalist endgame now playing out in subnational laboratories. Quite the contrary. Although the states as a whole are very much involved in health care policy, and a few may be closing in on broad reforms, only one (Hawaii) has approached affordable universal coverage and only two others (Washington and Minnesota) are now implementing legislation that may follow suit by the end of the decade. Five others (Florida, Massachusetts, Maryland, Vermont, and Oregon) have moved forcefully in that direction, but in these the commitment to universal coverage, affordability, or both remains in some doubt. The forty-two other denizens of the federal system have yet to devise firm plans to get everyone covered at prices likely to stay tolerable. Most states, therefore, are, so to speak, strategically challenged; for them, affordable universal coverage will be a dramatic departure.

Despite a celebrated surge of state activism in reforming health care in the past five years, affordable universal coverage has come hard for three reasons. For one thing, the states no more have a handy solution to tough financing questions than does the central government. Most flinch at medicaid's deepening bite on tax revenues, none has moved seriously toward a tax-financed universal system, and few want to fight employers over a mandate. Locked into competition with each other for a deeper tax base and new business, states find it as politically costly as Congress does—perhaps more so—to fund coverage for all.

Universal coverage has also been difficult to achieve because, as James

W. Fossett notes in chapter 3, few states have shown much enthusiasm for aggressive cost containment measures beyond their own immediate purview, medicaid. In a mixed public-private system each sector looks out for itself, so one would expect policymakers to launch systemwide efforts to curb spending only if private purchasers strongly pressure them to do so. Business, however, has almost everywhere been more inclined to bewail rising health costs than to demand government leadership in attacking them.[1] Amazingly, the states' record on cost containment in 1994 can be summed up in pretty much the same terms as in 1980. Setting of hospital rates by state agencies or commissions seems to work in the few states that have adopted and maintained rate-setting programs.

Third, sectoral segmentation has also inhibited the states' resolve to refashion the delivery system. Some states have promoted managed care for medicaid clients, and some businesses have urged managed care on their workers, but managed care has come to mean a motley array of payment, provider, and review systems, and these miscellaneous public and private initiatives have yet to meet in coherent statewide health policies. Likewise, as Michael Sparer points out in chapter 5, states have been slow to battle academic medical centers and the medical establishment to produce more general, or family, physicians and seldom come forward with enough money to induce medical workers to practice in underserved areas. And most states, Frank Thompson shows in chapter 4, have left experiments to improve the quality of care to the clinicians and economists crafting medical practice guidelines and outcome measures within federal precincts.

Although the states deserve credit for their policy innovations in the past five years, one should resist romanticizing their reach and grasp. For most the comprehensive, integrated, disciplined synthesis of universal coverage, cost control, and reform of the delivery system that is envisioned in the Clinton plan lies far beyond their ken, and the harmonious interaction of quality care, universal access, and program efficiency that reformers seek would be a dramatic departure from the status quo. Firm federal leadership would lighten the states' load. If the federal government established universal coverage, a basic benefit package, and a financing framework, these thorny issues would be lifted from the states' agendas. But if states were required to raise all or part of the money (as in a single-payer option) or to regulate an alliance-based system that defines the cost of employers' shares of workers' insurance premiums, they would still face conflict over financing issues, albeit in more focused form.

If the federal government set cost-growth targets for the states or for health alliance regions within them, states would perhaps have less to fear politically from providers—until the inevitable community conflicts over the reduction of services that could be required to stay within funding limits worked their way to the offices of governors and legislators. If the central government devised incentives that favored managed care, the reform of the delivery system would advance by the indirect and invisible hand of market forces—until providers and consumers, upset over new patterns of competition and their consequences for access and quality, began complaining that states were doing a poor job of certifying plans, monitoring their behavior, and fashioning correctives. All this is not to say that the states would not welcome a national plan or that they could not implement it successfully, but it does suggest that well-crafted federal innovation will complicate states' lives as much as ill-considered ones and that analysts and political leaders should not underestimate the magnitude of the reform project.

Steering a Reformed System: Five Undervalued Functions

Affordable universal coverage in the federal system will demand a new intergovernmental division of labor. Reallocating functions is difficult enough in theory and will be even more so in practice because each stratagem for a better balance among quality, access, and cost will create new occasions for credit claiming and blame shifting. The analyses in this book suggest that five tasks are especially important to workable state implementation of national health reform. But each, though fundamental, has tended to be relegated to the periphery of the health care debate.

Regulation

A reformed health care system will require a much enlarged public regulatory authority, perhaps to oversee the behavior of providers and patients, certainly to monitor budgets at both the national and state levels.[2] Leery of speaking plainly about regulation, policymakers have sought to make such activity inconspicuous by describing it as a "backstop" to be triggered only if the magic of the marketplace fails to work. It is most unlikely, however, that coverage can be made and kept affordable unless policy adds a potent new dose of macroregulation of systemwide budgets to the present microregulation of providers' behavior.

The Clinton plan's backstop would have the federal government set baseline and "year one" budgets that alliances and health plans must learn to live within. Although as a formal matter the states would be largely excused from participation in the ensuing conflicts, it is unlikely that they could stay aloof for long. And of course bargaining in Congress might well reject so large an augmentation of federal authority and send a diluted version to the states. As James Fossett observes in chapter 3, however, there is a big difference between a rate-setting system that covers only hospitals or the regulation of rates paid for medicare patients and the regulation of total health care expenditures. Neither the federal government nor the states have much institutional capacity for regulating revenues or insurance prices.

Regulatory challenges carry well beyond cost control, moreover. Truly universal private health care coverage demands new pools of purchasers and dramatic insurance reforms. It therefore requires firm rules defining the contributions that sustain the pools and measures to halt the selection of preferred risks. Secure, affordable private coverage also obliges states or regional pools to administer subsidies for individuals or businesses or perhaps both. If access is to improve, physicians cannot remain entirely free to specialize in whatever they wish and practice how and where they please. Either large and costly incentives must be offered or firm new rules must be invented to favor general practitioners and practices in underserved areas. If the federal or state governments (or both) decide to emphasize a formal agenda for improving quality of care, appropriate agencies must develop standards of practice, report cards, and other means of assessing and improving quality and then hold health plans accountable. As Frank Thompson notes in chapter 4, however, such innovations are as much a quantum leap beyond current regulatory practice for the federal government and the states as are the global revenue-constraining strategies proposed to supplement market forces.

The plausible contours of federal-state sharing of regulatory powers are far from clear. In principle the federal government might set broad performance standards or targets to which state implementers would be held accountable. But states do not want the politically dirty work of enforcing budget caps, work force quotas, or quality-improvement schemes hatched in Washington, which is one main reason why the Clinton plan assigns many of these activities to new national or regional boards or agencies. The prospect of new agencies, however, conjures up lurid visions of "new layers of federal bureaucracy," so it would not be strange if such regulatory authority as emerged were much weakened and parceled out ambiguously among federal, regional, and state bodies. Meanwhile, as James Fossett remarks in chapter 3, a long list of political stimuli—pressures from local entities that lose power or funding, the possibility of adverse judicial decisions and the need to make regulatory judgments that are defensible in court, uncertainties associated with important measurements, concerns about adequate access to care, quality of care, and risk selection, and more—will drive implementers to levels of regulatory specificity at which neither experience nor staff capacities have prepared them to operate.

Information

Regulators (or for that matter rational actors in reinvigorated markets) cannot steer the system accurately without detailed knowledge about what and how its components are doing. For this they need good and abundant data, the mother's milk of management. Generating and packaging such information is a major undertaking in itself. Health alliances need to know what health plans do to and for their enrollees, but battles may rage among them, the states, the plans, and consumer groups over what information must or should be made available to whom and who gets to interpret it. (The sharper the competition, presumably the sharper the conflict over the definition of proprietary information and the terms of its release.)

Those groups monitoring quality need extensive information on the use and clinical consequences of medical procedures. But the interpretation of these data is as much administrative art as it is clinical science. Frank Thompson notes that policymakers' aggressive promotion of quality faces enormous methodological problems, including the application of controls for variables that complicate the surface relation between medical acts and outcomes and the risk that plans may polish their quality profiles by shifting resources from unmeasured procedures to those that are highlighted in report cards. New patterns in the health care work force should rest on information that links demographic trends and community resources to patterns of specialization and location. Cost containment presupposes timely and extensive data on who is spending what, where, and for what groups over time.

In one sense such data are disturbingly plentiful. But, as James Fossett comments, the large number of payers, the limited agreement on standards for data, and deep incompatibilities between forms, software, and other system particulars makes developing standard measures an expensive, difficult, and lengthy job. The regulation of revenues and spending is extremely data intensive, and the necessary information infrastructure is mostly absent. Filling the gaps means sophisticated computer systems, more numerous and better trained staff to gather and analyze data, and, of course, the money to build these capacities. How far such measures erase the administrative savings alleged to follow from standardized benefits, electronic paper flows, and other innovations is an intriguing question. Be that as it may, the federal and state governments would improve the prospects for implementation by investing significantly in better managers and management information systems now. But because such improvements are invisible to the public, politicians often give them short shrift.

Planning

Planning cowers alongside rationing and taxing in the lexicon of expletives deleted from the debate on health care reform. Market forces will trigger all the planning one needs within health care plans themselves; overt governmental planning need not apply. Yet many demands on and for public planning are implicit in health reform. If markets are to be reorganized into large purchasing pools, some public authority must define the pools and their area boundaries in ways that produce an equitable (or at any rate politically sustainable) allocation of risks and costs. If all citizens are to have a choice of good quality health plans in their communities, including poor inner cities and remote rural areas, some overseer must make certain that service capacity, and the right kind of capacity, is there. Such assurances, taken seriously, define a long planning agenda. Perhaps health plans can be required to serve Bedford-Stuyvesant and Wyoming, but can they be required to serve them well? How, and by whose standards? Will the "efficient" plans expected to manage everyone's care also take the trouble to plan and manage the integration of medical and social services for vulnerable populations with special needs? If plans resist helping to salvage "essential community providers," will states plan how, and how far, to keep them in business? If, as is likely, medicare beneficiaries, veterans, prisoners, and undocumented aliens remain outside the reformed system, will states plan for the ensuing fiscal and institutional "interfaces"?

Quality assurance demands reliable systems for appraising the clinical utility (and cost effectiveness) of existing medical procedures and those emerging from the research pipeline—and for deploying this information in ways that empower consumers. States then must plan how to get consumers to use the report cards and kindred information. As Michael Sparer shows in chapter 5, gauging the nation's need for nurses and physicians is no simple matter. Planning wrong could mean an oversupply of generalists or specialists, too few providers caring adequately for the poor, or continuing geographic maldistribution. The interplay of demographic trends, population movements, financial pressures on institutions, and organizational adaptations and reconfigurations (for example, integrated services networks) regularly wreaks havoc on estimates of community and regional needs. Cost containment requires realistic projections of who can cut what for whom and how fast, lest clumsy squeezing generate underservice or inferior quality for portions of the population or economic failures and local chaos that upsets communities and consumers.

Planning is the flip side of information—the managerial use of information systems to anticipate from present data what seems to be coming next and what that may mean for policy goals. Such planning is intrinsically hard, harder in a private-centered system that consigns government to the roles of catalyst and constrainer, and hardest when (as now) it has no constituency. But without improved federal and state capacities to plan, to discern trends and make adjustments that steer the system reliably, the desired new equilibrium among quality, access, and cost may not be realized or may not hold for long.

Negotiation

Invisible market hands and government backstopping regulations will not work well unless the parties at interest can negotiate their conflicts. Pluralism notwithstanding, negotiating machinery is difficult to build into implementation frameworks in the United States. The Right deplores the implied affirmation of the authority of the government "side," while the Left fears that interest group liberalism will rear its ugly head if the governmental lamb lies down with the lions. But if employers and consumers do not like the way the health alliances work, they must be able to complain constructively to someone—presumably a state or national agency. Many complex issues of governance and representation that define the numbers, roles, and powers of employers and consumers on health alliance boards must be settled if pooled purchasing is to work smoothly. If health plans, their provider components, disease groups, or others with a stake in monitoring quality and the design of report cards take issue with the development or use of regulatory methods, they need reliable channels of communication. Frank Thompson suggests in chapter 4 that responsibility for negotiating specifications for report cards, and the conflicts that go with the job, might best be given to the states, but, citing the surprisingly protracted process by which New York State reached agreement with health maintenance organizations over such measures, he also warns that negotiations will be difficult and slow. The institutions that train medical personnel and the communities that prefer one or another work force mix will want to explain how policy changes could affect them. Health plans struggling to adapt to new cost-containing regulations may seek a dialogue with those setting and enforcing limits so that implementation is not principally played out in the media, the courts, and the legislature. Likewise, plans that do not develop sturdy bargaining provisions for their physicians and providers may be undone by internal conflict as they search for market security.

Regulatory rulings handed down from above, even as backstops, will be hard to implement in a health care system as community centered and averse to government intrusion as the one in the United States. Loyalty (political deference and commitment to the reform "cause") is weak, and exit is not an option in a comprehensively reformed system, so the demand for an effective voice looms very large.[3] Other societies seem to address this need better, ironically, than does the ostentatiously participatory United States.

At some point down the long evolutionary road to reform, the health care system will be obliged to marry regional and local preferences about access and quality with significant state or federal limits on the flow of funds into the health care system. In the 1970s health systems agencies were expected to test these waters, but funding limits were not adopted and the agencies lacked regulatory power. In the 1980s policymakers hoped that managed care and competition would discipline the system, but these merely aggravated its wanton ways. In the early 1990s health alliances were sold as the latest best hope, but these too seem to be fading fast. There remains a vast institutional chasm that will eventually be bridged, but by means as yet indistinct. Very likely the community level is too small and self-regarding to house such institutional machinery, the federal government too remote and distrusted, and regions too artificial—all of which points toward new and as yet inchoate roles for the states as political foci for the planning and negotiating structures that will in due course emerge.

Reorganization

As policy debates explore the benefits and costs to be conferred on or withdrawn from myriad interested parties, the organization of the public authorities that will implement the new regime understandably stays on the sidelines of public discourse. Yet reform will mean new demands for regulation, information, planning, and negotiation, and these will not find easy accommodation within existing state organizations at work on health care affairs. Affordable universal coverage will compel states to tackle tasks that their departments of health, social services, insurance, and others will find unfamiliar and perhaps alien. States buy health insurance for their employees and for medicaid clients, and some have established sizable public purchasing pools, but none has worked with the immense health alliances envisioned in the Clinton plan or in other versions of managed competition, and none has confronted the conflicts that will arise over the economic distributions and redistributions that pooled jurisdictions would create.

States certify health plans but not with the close eye on relations among access, quality, and cost that affordable universal coverage demands. Nor do they focus on the requisites of fiscal solvency in an environment of constrained resources. Some have embraced insurance reform, but none has yet tried to enforce the whole package, including portability, community rating, limits on exclusions for preexisting conditions, and related deterrents to preferred-risk selection. States control licensing and include quality as one element in their regulatory decisions, but they have little experience with the ambitious measures of process and outcome that report cards and related monitoring schemes anticipate. As Michael Sparer remarks in chapter 5, in most states policy toward the work force is a loosely coordinated product of distinct medical and educational "tracks," and few states have adopted more than modest programs to aid the inner cities and the underserved in rural areas. Many have struggled to slow the growth of medical spending by means of fee schedules and managed care, but state agencies' experience with spending or revenue caps mainly ends with hospitals. And few states have shown much taste even for that.

As one contemplates implementation of a health care plan, administrative questions jump out from all sides. What agencies, old or new, are best equipped for these tasks, and what would be their division of labor? What staff skills and numbers will they need to perform these functions, and what new funds, data, training, and authority will the staffs require? What demands on interagency cooperation will affordable universal coverage impose? That there are no easy or evident answers to these questions is true enough but beside the present point, which is that these questions are too seldom aired and explicated.

Politics and Administration

It is one thing to identify gaps in states' implementation capacities, and quite another to marshal the resources to fill them. Implementing program details and managing institutional complexity are far down the list of priorities of most of those promoting health reform. If market forces are in vogue as an antidote to big government, who wants to advertise the extensive public management required to make markets serve the public interest? Similarly, those who favor public-centered solutions such as a single-payer system anticipate a large reduction in the administrative costs and conundrums that now accompany private health insurance and show little patience for discussing how to improve public administration in a system that leaves private insurance in place, albeit constrained. Management issues are not, prima facie, about the allocation of clinical or economic benefits and costs; they address the doings not of caregivers and policy leaders but of public officials. These issues and officials have scarcely any constituency and therefore command little sympathetic attention. When policy goes awry, however, they get plenty of attention, little of it sympathetic.

It is hardly profound to propose that states are likely to perform the tasks of regulation, information collection and dissemination, planning, negotiation, and reorganization more credibly if state political leaders recognize their importance and commit money and time to helping the administrative apparatus charged with implementing change. There is, however, no good reason to expect that very many state leaders will do so. Adding, trimming, and rearranging bureaucratic units and functions and spending more on administrative infrastructure do not resonate well with most contestants in a debate about how to shrink costs and broaden benefits. And policymakers have trouble explaining administrative reasoning to an electorate that is at once impatient for change and skeptical that any version of it government delivers up will serve the public interest. It does not help that relations between policy ends and managerial means are highly speculative in all the major reform alternatives.

Intergovernmental tensions further complicate state leaders' political calculations. Neither state administrators nor their political bosses will invest effort and resources in improving management if their hands are tied tightly by federal rules that oblige them to act contrary to their preferences or prohibit behavior that makes sense to them. States have complained for years about the federal government's readiness to impose mandates and its reluctance to grant waivers from difficult requirements.[4] On the one hand, a stream of national impositions, often unaccompanied by adequate federal funding, in such programs as medicaid unsettles state budgets and complicates administrative lives. On the other hand, federal interpretations of medicare, medicaid, Employee Retirement Income Security Act (ERISA), and the tax treatment of health benefits limit state options for reform. And the obstacles to waiving these requirements have deterred many would-be innovators. (The fate of ERISA and other waivers sought by Washington, Minnesota, Florida, and others remains to be seen.)

Although some may attribute the intergovernmental frustrations of the mandate-waiver syndrome to poor performance in the federal bureaucracy, the buck does not stop there. Bureaucratic politics in federal health agencies unfolds amidst larger political storms perpetually swirling around the legislative-executive politics of health care in Washington. Health care policy evokes intense conflicts over values and interests, and the institutional character of the policy machinery makes consensus and coalition building difficult. In the inevitable uphill search for legislative agreement, strategies that violate the "rules" of a sound intergovernmental compact often prove expedient. Giving states broad flexibility to implement policy while holding them accountable to outcome or performance standards may make good administrative sense, but in practice, detailed provisions requiring or prohibiting one or another pattern of state behavior can win the votes of legislators who distrust the ideological or partisan proclivities of state regimes or who simply fear loss of federal control. Spelling out clearly the scope of state duties and the terms of federal delegation is advisable in theory, but adopting vague and elliptical statutory language ("the states shall address x or y in a plan to be devised subject to regulations to be issued by the Secretary of Health and Human Services") on points of contention that threaten coalitions can win supporters, and at the seemingly minor price of devolving to the states some of the toughest decisions about policy.

The politics of federal policymaking often defeat orderly federalism and regularly confer in the states the worst of both worlds—tight federal constraints that inhibit innovation and responsiveness plus broad delegations of authority that expect states to solve problems that send federal leaders running for political cover. These patterns go with the territory of U.S. policymaking, but their costs are considerable. They reduce the incentives of state political leaders to grapple with health care policy and try to sustain legislative and managerial innovation; dim leaders' willingness to support administrative improvements; and give public managers the impression that coherence and effectiveness in their spheres are not necessarily expected, noticed, and rewarded. This debilitating interplay among politics, policy, and administration is neither accidental nor easily corrected. Analysis and discussion are far from sufficient to set matters right. But they are probably necessary to contain political costs that cannot be entirely avoided and to improve the quality of health care policy in an inherently disorderly intergovernmental milieu.

Notes

Introduction

1. Herbert Kaufman, *The Forest Ranger: A Study in Administrative Behavior* (Johns Hopkins Press, 1960), p. 3.

2. Drew E. Altman and Douglas H. Morgan, "The Role of State and Local Government in Health," *Health Affairs*, vol. 2 (Winter 1983), pp. 7–31.

3. Ibid., pp. 8–9.

4. Based on a presentation by W. David Helms, conference on "Health Care Reform and the Role of the States," Institute of Government and Public Affairs, University of Chicago, April 29, 1994.

5. Richard P. Nathan, "The Role of the States in American Federalism," in Carl Van Horn, ed., *The State of the States* (Washington: Congressional Quarterly Press, 1989), pp. 17–18.

6. Woodrow Wilson, *Constitutional Government in the United States* (Columbia University Press, 1908; reprinted 1961), p. 173.

7. Martha Derthick, *Agency under Stress: The Social Security Administration in American Government* (Brookings, 1990), p. 4.

Chapter One

1. General Accounting Office, *Medicare Claims*, GAO/HR-93-6 (December 1992).

2. Michael Sparer and Lawrence D. Brown, "Between a Rock and a Hard Place: How Public Managers Manage Medicaid," in Frank J. Thompson, ed., *Revitalizing State and Local Public Service: Strengthening Performance, Accountability, and Citizen Confidence* (San Francisco: Jossey-Bass, 1993), pp. 279–306.

3. Donald F. Kettl, *Government by Proxy: (Mis?)Managing Federal Programs* (Congressional Quarterly Press, 1988); Richard Nathan, *Turning Promise into Performance* (Columbia University Press, 1993); and John J. DiIulio, Jr., Gerald Garvey, and Donald F. Kettl, *Improving Government Performance: An Owner's Manual* (Brookings, 1993).

4. Congressional Budget Office, *An Analysis of the Administration's Health Proposal* (1994), p. 15.

5. General Accounting Office, *Health Insurance Regulation: Wide Variation in States' Authority, Oversight, and Resources*, HRD-94-26 (December 1993).

6. General Accounting Office, *Information Management and Technology Issues*, OCG-93-5TR (December 1992), p. 4.

7. "Health Care Reform at Risk," *New York Times*, March 27, 1994, sec. 4, p. 16.

8. GAO, *Information Management and Technology Issues*, p. 10.

9. See National Commission on the State and Local Public Service, *Frustrated Federalism: Rx for State and Local Health Care Reform* (Albany: Nelson A. Rockefeller Institute of Government, 1993), esp. chap. 7.

10. Melvina Ford and others, *Summary Comparison of Major Health Care Reform Bills* (Congressional Research Service, January 6, 1994).

11. "Consumer Choice Health Security Act: Fact Sheet," U.S. Senate, November 20, 1993.

Chapter Two

1. William A. Glaser, *Health Insurance in Practice* (San Francisco: Jossey-Bass, 1991).

2. W. David Helms and others, "Mending the Flaws in the Small-Group Market," and Catherine G. McLaughlin and Wendy K. Zellers, "Shortcomings of Voluntarism in the Small-Group Market," *Health Affairs*, vol. 11 (Summer 1992), pp. 7–27, 28–40; and Wendy K. Zellers and others, "Small-Business Health Insurance: Only Healthy Need Apply," *Health Affairs*, vol. 11 (Spring 1992), pp. 174–80.

3. On the development of alliances and other elements of managed competition, see Alain C. Enthoven, "The History and Principles of Managed Competition," *Health Affairs*, vol. 12 (Supplement 1993), pp. 24–48. On the Jackson Hole group, see John Hubner, "The Abandoned Father of Health-Care Reform," *New York Times Magazine*, July 18, 1993, p. 24.

4. The text of President Clinton's Health Security Act is presented and summarized in Commerce Clearing House, *President Clinton's Health Care Reform Proposal: Health Security Act: CCH Professional Summary and Text of Bill* (Chicago: Commerce Clearing House, 1993). State responsibilities are discussed on pp. 52–54, alliances on pp. 54–61. See also National Academy of Social Insurance, *The President's Proposal for Health Care Reform: An Overview of the Administrative Structure* (Washington: National Academy of Social Insurance, 1994), pp. 18–26.

5. Paul Starr, "Alliances for Progress," *New York Times*, March 6, 1994, sec. 4, p. 15.

6. Robert E. Patricelli, "Why Do We Need Health Alliances?" *Health Affairs*, vol. 13 (Spring 1994), pp. 239–42.

7. James T. O'Connor, "Flaw in Alliances," letter to editor, *New York Times*, March 17, 1994, p. A22.

8. On Maine's tribulations in designing small business subsidies in a voluntary program, see Lawrence D. Brown, "Policy Reform as Creative Destruction: Political and Administrative Challenges in Preserving the Public-Private Mix," *Inquiry*, vol. 29 (Summer 1992), pp. 189–90.

9. Congressional Budget Office, *An Analysis of the Administration's Health Proposal* (February 1994), pp. 17–18.

10. DeAnn Friedholm, in *Implementing a Reformed Health Care System: The View from the Field*, transcript of conference held at the Nelson A. Rockefeller Institute of Government, Albany, November 1993, p. 63.

11. For a lucid review of governance issues and options, see Walter A. Zelman, "Who Should Govern the Purchasing Cooperative?" *Health Affairs*, vol. 12 (Supplement 1993), pp. 49–57.

12. CBO, *Administration's Health Proposal*, p. 70.

13. Ibid., p. 73.

14. Margaret Stanley, in *Implementing a Reformed Health Care System*, pp. 60–61.

15. Margaret T. Stanley, "Controlling Health Costs and Expanding Access to Care: The Value of Purchasing Cooperatives," statement to the Subcommittee on Health and Environment and Subcommittee on Commerce, Consumer Protection, and Competitiveness, November 2, 1993, p. 4.

16. David Maxwell-Jolly, in *Implementing a Reformed Health Care System*, pp. 21–22.

17. On CALPERS see General Accounting Office, *California Public Employees' Alliance Has Reduced Recent Premium Growth*, HRD 94-40 (November 1993).

18. For background on Florida and Washington, see Lawrence D. Brown, "Commissions, Clubs, and Consensus: Florida Reorganizes for Health Reform," and Robert A. Crittenden, "Managed Competition and Premium Caps in Washington State," *Health Affairs*, vol. 12 (Summer 1993), pp. 7–26, 82–88.

Chapter Three

1. See, for example, the defense of the administration's premium caps offered in Richard Kronick, "A Helping Hand for the Invisible Hand," *Health Affairs*, vol. 13 (Spring 1994), pp. 96–101; and David Rogers, "House Panel Splits over Cost Controls in Health Plan," *Wall Street Journal*, March 11, 1994, p. A2.

2. Lawrence D. Brown, "Commissions, Clubs, and Consensus: Florida Reorganizes for Health Reform," *Health Affairs*, vol. 12 (Summer 1993), pp. 7–26.

3. See Joseph White, *Competing Solutions: American Health Care Proposals and International Experience* (Brookings, forthcoming), chap. 8, for an excellent brief description of these rules.

4. See Rogers, "House Panel Splits," p. A2.

5. For one example of such claims, see Richard Kronick, "Helping Hand," p. 100.

6. Alain C. Enthoven and Sara J. Singer, "A Single-Payer System in Jackson Hole Clothing," and Mark V. Pauly, "The Clinton Plan: What Happened to the Tough Choices?" *Health Affairs*, vol. 13 (Spring 1994), pp. 85, 147–60.

7. Price Waterhouse, Washington National Tax Services, "Premium Growth Targets under the Clinton Proposal: Comparison with the OECD Experience," October 1993.

8. John Iglehart, "The American Health Care System: Managed Care," *New England Journal of Medicine*, September 3, 1992, pp. 742–47.

9. Congressional Budget Office, "The Effects of Managed Care on Use and Costs of Health Services," staff memorandum, June 1992.

10. Iglehart, "American Health Care System," p. 743.

11. Clive S. Thomas and Ronald J. Hrebenar, "Interest Groups in the States," in Virginia Gray, Herbert Jacob, and Robert B. Albritton, eds., *Politics in the American States: A Comparative Analysis*, 4th ed. (Scott Foresman, 1990), pp. 123–58.

12. See CBO, "The Effects of Managed Care on Use and Cost of Health Care Services"; and Congressional Budget Office, *The Potential Impact of Certain Forms of Managed Care on Health Care Expenditures* (August 1992). See also William B. Schwartz and Daniel N. Mendelson, "Why Managed Care Cannot Contain Hospital Costs—Without Rationing," *Health Affairs*, vol. 11 (Summer 1992), pp. 100–08.

13. Alain C. Enthoven, "Why Managed Care Has Failed to Contain Health Costs," *Health Affairs*, vol. 12 (Fall 1993), pp. 27–43.

14. See, for example, Walter A. Zelman, "The Rationale behind the Clinton Health Reform Plan," *Health Affairs*, vol. 13 (Spring 1994), pp. 9–29.

15. Elizabeth Kilbreath and Alan Cohen, "Strategic Choices for Cost Containment under a Reformed U.S. Health Care System," *Inquiry*, vol. 30 (Winter 1993), pp. 372–88.

16. Iglehart, "American Health Care System," pp. 742–47.

17. See, for example, Alain C. Enthoven and Richard Kronick, "A Consumer Choice Health Plan for the 1990's: Universal Health Insurance in a System Designed to Promote Quality and Economy," *New England Journal of Medicine*, January 5, 1989, pp. 29–37, and January 12, 1989, pp. 94–101; Kilbreath and Cohen, "Strategic Choices," pp. 376–77; and Congressional Budget Office, *Managed Competition and Its Potential to Reduce Health Spending* (May 1993), p. 40.

18. Richard Kronick and others, "The Market Place in Health Care Reform: The Demographic Limitations of Managed Competition," *New England Journal of Medicine*, January 14, 1993, pp. 148–52.

19. Paul P. Cooper III and Kylanne Green, "The Impact of State Laws on Managed Care," *Health Affairs*, vol. 10 (Winter 1991), pp. 161–69.

20. "A Sneak Attack on Health Reform," *New York Times*, April 11, 1994, p. A18.

21. A useful framework for these issues is provided in Kenneth Cahill and others, "Prospective Budgeting for Medicare Physician Service" (Congressional Research Service, 1989).

22. William A. Glaser, "How Expenditure Caps and Targets Really Work," *Milbank Quarterly*, vol. 71 (1993), pp. 97–127, provides a useful inventory of current practice.

23. Gerard F. Anderson, "All-Payer Ratesetting: Down but Not Out," *Health Care Financing Review* (1991 annual supplement), pp. 35–41.

24. Congressional Budget Office, *Responses to Uncompensated Care and Public-Program Controls on Spending: Do Hospitals Cost Shift?* (May 1993).

25. The most visible of these experiments has been in Rochester, New York. For accounts, see William J. Hall and Paul F. Griner, "Cost-Effective Health Care: The Rochester Experience," *Health Affairs*, vol. 12 (Spring 1993), pp. 58–69; and Sara E. Hartman and Dana B. Mukamel, "How Might a Low-Cost Hospital System Look?" *Medical Care*, vol. 27 (March 1989), pp. 234–43.

26. Congressional Budget Office, *Medicare's Disproportionate Share Adjustments for Hospitals* (May 1990), pp. 42–43.

27. Kenneth E. Thorpe, "Health Care," in Gerald Benjamin and Charles Brecher, eds., *The Two New Yorks: State-City Relations in the Changing Federal System* (Russell Sage, 1988);

and Kevin Volpp and Bruce Siegel, "New Jersey: Long Term Experience with All-Payer State Rate Setting," *Health Affairs*, vol. 12 (Summer 1993), pp. 59–66.

28. Anderson, "All-Payer Ratesetting," p. 36.

29. Robert Hackey, "Trapped between State and Market: Regulating Hospital Reimbursement in the Northeastern States," *Medical Care Review*, vol. 49 (Fall 1992), pp. 355–88; and interviews with officials of the Office of Health Systems Management.

30. For evidence on the effects of state schemes, see Anderson, "All-Payer Ratesetting," pp. 35–41; Kenneth E. Thorpe, "The American States and Canada: A Comparative Analysis of Health Care Spending," *Journal of Health Politics, Policy and Law*, vol. 18 (Summer 1993), pp. 477–91; and Hackey, "Trapped between State and Market."

31. The enormous literature on medicare's PPS scheme is summarized in Robert Coulam and Gary Gaumier, "Medicare's Prospective Payment System: A Critical Appraisal," *Health Care Financing Review* (1991 annual supplement), pp. 45–77.

32. See Glaser, "How Expenditure Caps and Targets Really Work"; and Bradford L. Kirkman-Liff, "Physician Payment and Cost Containment in West Germany: Suggestions for Medicare Reform," *Journal of Health Politics, Policy and Law*, vol. 15 (Spring 1990), pp. 69–101.

33. Ian Ayres and John Braithwaite, *Responsive Regulation: Transcending the Deregulation Debate* (Oxford University Press, 1992); and Ayres and Braithwaite, "Tripartism: Regulatory Capture and Empowerment," *Law and Social Inquiry* (1991), pp. 435–96.

34. The best description of this process is contained in Congressional Budget Office, *An Analysis of the Administration's Health Proposal* (February 1994), pp. 22–23.

35. Margaret Stanley and Nan Schroeder, in *Implementing a Reformed Health Care System: The View from the Field*, transcript of conference held at the Nelson A. Rockefeller Institute of Government, Albany, November 1993, pp. 172, 185; and Robert A. McGuire, Brian W. Tvenstrup, and Jeremy E. Roller, "Implementing Health Reform: A Three-State Analysis of the Clinton Plan," Woodrow Wilson School, Princeton University, 1994.

36. Zelman, "Rationale behind the Clinton Health Reform Plan."

37. This argument is made most efficiently in Charles L. Schultze, *The Public Use of Private Interest* (Brookings, 1977), pp. 21–25. See also Enthoven, "Why Managed Care Has Failed to Contain Health Care Costs."

38. See Paul Starr, "Design of Health Insurance Purchasing Cooperatives," and Walter A. Zelman, "Who Should Govern the Purchasing Cooperative?" *Health Affairs*, vol. 12 (supplement 1993), pp. 49–57, 58–64.

39. This discussion of Federal Reserve operations relies heavily on John Woolley, *Monetary Politics: The Federal Reserve Bank and the Politics of Monetary Policy* (Cambridge University Press, 1984).

40. The most prominent of these accounts are Edward R. Tufte, *Political Control of the Economy* (Princeton University Press, 1978); and William D. Nordhaus, "The Political Business Cycle," *Review of Economic Studies*, vol. 42 (April 1975), pp. 169–90.

41. Woolley, *Monetary Politics*, p. 193.

42. Ibid., p. 152.

43. This section relies on Carol Ebdon, "The Military Base Closing Commission: A Case Study in Politics and Administration," State University of New York–Albany, Department of Public Administration and Policy, 1993.

44. Mike Mills, "Base Closings: The Political Pain Is Limited," *Congressional Quarterly Weekly Report*, December 31, 1988, pp. 3625–29.

45. Robert A. Caro, *The Power Broker: Robert Moses and the Fall of New York* (Knopf, 1974).

46. For a useful, if somewhat lurid, description of these agencies, see Donald Axelrod, *Shadow Government* (Wiley, 1992).

47. For a useful comparison of the two states, see Hackey, "Trapped between State and Market."

48. See, for example, Bruce A. Williams, "Regulation and Economic Development," in Gray, Jacob, and Albritton, eds., *Politics in the American States: A Comparative Analysis*, pp. 479–523.

49. See, for example, James A. Morone and Andrew B. Dunham, "Slouching Toward National Health Insurance: The New Health Care Politics," *Yale Journal of Regulation*, vol. 2 (1985), pp. 263–91; Hackey, "Trapped between State and Market"; and Lawrence D. Brown, "Political Evolution of Health Care Regulation," *Health Affairs*, vol. 11 (Winter 1992), pp. 17–37.

50. *United Wire, Metal and Machine Health and Welfare Fund* v. *Morristown Memorial Hospital et al.*, 793 F. Supp. 524 (D. N.J. 1992); and *Travelers Insurance Company* v. *Cuomo et al.* and *Health Insurance Association of America* v. *Chassin et al.*, 813 F. Supp. 996 (S.D. N.Y. 1993).

51. See Gerard F. Anderson and Mark A. Hall, "The Adequacy of Hospital Reimbursement under Medicaid's Boren Amendment," *Journal of Legal Medicine*, vol. 13 (1992), pp. 205–36, for a discussion of recent litigation.

52. *Clark* v. *Kizer*, 758 F. Supp. 572 (E.D. Cal. 1990); decided in court of appeals as *Clark* v. *Coye*, 8 F.3d 26 (9th Cir. 1993).

53. See Mark A. Hall and Gerard F. Anderson, "Health Insurers' Assessment of Medical Necessity," *University of Pennsylvania Law Review*, vol. 140 (May 1992), pp. 1637–1712; and George Anders, "More Insurers Pay for Care That's in Trials," *Wall Street Journal*, February 15, 1994, pp. B1, B6.

54. The literature on these requirements and their judicial application in particular cases is vast, but a useful brief summary of the requirements is provided in Stephen Breyer, *Regulation and Its Reform* (Harvard University Press, 1982), app. 2.

55. See Enthoven and Singer, "Single-Payer System," p. 87.

56. Richard B. Stewart, "The Discontents of Legalism: Interest Group Relations in Administrative Regulation," *Wisconsin Law Review* (1985), pp. 655–86.

57. Robert T. Nakamura, Philip J. Cooper, and Thomas W. Church, Jr., "Environmental Dispute Resolution and Hazardous Waste Cleanups: A Cautionary Tale of Policy Implementation," *Journal of Policy Analysis and Management*, vol. 10 (Spring 1991), pp. 204–22.

58. Physician Payment Review Commission, *Annual Report to Congress, 1990*, appendix D.

59. Katherine R. Levitt and others, "Health Spending by State: New Estimates for Policy Making," *Health Affairs*, vol. 12 (Fall 1993), p. 8.

60. Physician Payment Review Commission, *Annual Report 1992*, chap. 10.

61. Ann Cherlow and others, "Data Quality in the Medicaid Statistical Information System (MSIS)" (SysteMetrics/McGraw-Hill, December 1991). See also General Accounting

Office, *Medicaid: Data Improvements Needed to Help Manage Health Care Program*, ITMEC-93-18 (May 1993).

62. Deborah Lewis-Idema, *Monitoring Medicaid Provider Participation and Access to Care* (Washington: National Governors' Association Health Policy Studies, 1992).

63. Physician Payment Review Commission, *Annual Report 1992*, chap. 10; and General Accounting Office, *Automated Medical Records: Leadership Needed to Expedite Standards Development*, ITMEC-93-17 (April 1993).

64. For a description of this system, see Minnesota Department of Health, *Minnesota Integrated Data Initiative to Support Health Care Reform: Preliminary Data Collection Plan* (St. Paul, 1993).

65. See Joseph P. Newhouse, "Patients at Risk: Health Reform and Risk Adjustment," *Health Affairs* (Spring 1994), pp. 132–46; and CBO, *Analysis of the Administration's Health Proposal*.

66. National Health Policy Forum, "The Price of No Data: Setting Private Insurance Premiums for the Uninsured," issue brief 644, 1994.

67. See Breyer, *Regulation and Its Reform*, chaps. 2 and 5, for a discussion and examples.

68. This dispute is chronicled in Thomas R. Oliver, "Analysis, Advice, and Congressional Leadership: The Physician Payment Review Commission and the Politics of Medicare," *Journal of Health Politics, Policy and Law*, vol. 18 (Spring 1993), pp. 113–75.

69. Comment from DeAnn Friedholm to author.

70. Breyer, *Regulation and Its Reform*, p. 179.

71. I am indebted to Jim Tallon for the distinction in this paragraph.

Chapter Four

1. *Politics* carries no invidious connotation as used here. The jockeying for influence over administrative decisions by various players can ventilate important views and yield constructive outcomes. Like other forms of politics, the bureaucratic variant can serve noble or ignoble ends.

2. Five other reform bills under consideration in 1994 (McDermott-Wellstone, Michel-Lott, Cooper-Breaux, Stearns-Nickles, Thomas-Chafee) vary greatly in the attention they pay to quality assurance. See Melvina Ford and others, *Summary Comparison of Major Health Care Reform Bills* (Congressional Research Service, January 6, 1994.)

3. White House Domestic Policy Council, *Health Security: The President's Report to the American People* (Washington: September 9, 1983), p. 100.

4. Data furnished by the American Association of Medical Colleges.

5. State licensure activities have, for instance, drawn criticism. An estimated 28,000 unlicensed persons are practicing medicine in the United States. See Paul Jesilow, Henry N. Pontell, and Gilbert Geis, *Prescription for Profit* (University of California Press, 1993), p. 198. Others note that most states have failed to expand licensure to freestanding facilities, such as those involved in cardiac catheterization, testing of blood samples, and radiation therapy for cancer. See General Accounting Office, *Limited State Efforts to Assure Quality of Care outside Hospitals*, HRD-90-53 (January 1990). The Citizen Advocacy Center in Washington, D.C., has documented many of the infirmities in state licensure activities. See, for instance, *A Resource Guide for Responding to Attempts to Weaken State Medical Licensing Boards*

by Legislating a Higher Standard of Evidence (Washington: Citizen Advocacy Center, October 1992).

6. Gary Clarke, in *Implementing a Reformed Health Care System: The View from the Field*, transcript of conference held at the Nelson A. Rockefeller Institute of Government, Albany, November 1993, p. 227. For a review of various definitions of quality, see R. Heather Palmer, Avedis Donabedian, and Gail J. Povar, *Striving for Quality in Health Care* (Ann Arbor, Mich.: Health Administration Press, 1991); and Office of Technology Assessment, *The Quality of Medical Care: Information for Consumers* (1988), pp. 53–55.

7. OTA, *Quality of Medical Care*, p. 9.

8. Donald L. Zimmerman, "Grading the Graders: Using 'Report Cards' to Enhance the Quality of Care under Health Care Reform," *National Health Policy Forum Issue Brief 642* (Washington: George Washington University, 1994).

9. Several reform plans in addition to the Clinton plan call for obtaining better information on the performance of medical providers. For instance, the Cooper-Breaux proposal calls for health care purchasing cooperatives to conduct enrollee satisfaction surveys and monitor disenrollment patterns in plans. The Thomas-Chafee bill would require plans to provide data on health outcomes and other indicators. Ford and others, *Summary Comparison*.

10. White House Domestic Policy Council, *Health Security*, p. 62.

11. Commerce Clearing House, *President Clinton's Health Care Reform Proposal: Health Security Act: CCH Professional Summary and Text of Bill* (Chicago: Commerce Clearing House, 1993), p. 246. The description of the national quality management council that follows is taken from this document, pp. 62, 246, 449–51, 455–57.

12. David Maxwell-Jolly, in *Implementing a Reformed Health Care System*, pp. 267–68.

13. New York State Department of Health, *Cardiac Surgery in New York State* (December 1993).

14. Ray Sweeney, in *Implementing a Reformed Health Care System*, p. 235.

15. David Maxwell-Jolly, in ibid., p. 269.

16. Ibid., p. 268.

17. Thomas Fanning, in ibid., pp. 73–74. In early 1994, the American Medical Association began meeting with representatives of hospitals, managed-care plans, and others to formulate a strategy to curtail proposed government efforts to collect health care data. See Barry Meier, "Hurdles Await Efforts to Rate Doctors and Medical Centers," *New York Times*, March 31, 1994, p. B8.

18. *Implementing a Reformed Health Care System*, p. 259.

19. Ibid., pp. 237–38.

20. Ray Sweeney, in ibid., p. 239.

21. Ibid., p. 247.

22. OTA, *Quality of Medical Care*, pp. 38, 44.

23. For a capsule overview of progress being made in the development of quality indicators, see "Let the (Quality-Based) Competition Begin!" *Rand Research Review*, vol. 17 (Winter 1993-94), pp. 1–3, 9.

24. I am indebted to Henry Aaron for drawing this point to my attention.

25. Among the alternative proposals, the McDermott-Wellstone plan speaks directly to the need for outcomes research and practice guidelines. Ford and others, *Summary Comparison*.

26. Walsh McDermott, "Evaluating the Physician and His Technology," in John H. Knowles, ed., *Doing Better and Feeling Worse: Health in the United States* (Norton, 1977), p. 143.

27. Stephen C. Schoenbaum, "Toward Fewer Procedures and Better Outcomes," *Journal of the American Medical Association*, February 10, 1993, p. 796.

28. John A. Wennberg, "AHCPR and the Strategy for Health Care Reform," *Health Affairs*, vol. 11 (Winter 1992), p. 67, 71.

29. Bradford H. Gray, "The Legislative Battle over Health Services Research," *Health Affairs*, vol. 11 (Winter 1992), pp. 38–66. AHCPR replaced the National Center for Health Services Research and Health Care Technology Assessment.

30. See General Accounting Office, *Practice Guidelines: The Experience of Medical Specialty Societies*, PEMD-91-11 (February 1991); and David M. Eddy, "Practice Policies: Where Do They Come From?" *Journal of the American Medical Association*, March 2, 1990, pp. 1265–75.

31. Utilization review typically features analysis of insurance claims to determine whether the care provided was "appropriate" and should be reimbursed. Utilization review can be prospective in that providers must obtain permission from the payer to perform certain procedures. Profile monitoring tends to be less immediately linked to payment. It often focuses on abstracts of hospital admissions and discharges to determine which providers are outliers in terms of the frequency with which they perform certain medical procedures. These outliers may then be subject to more careful scrutiny, comment, and even sanction.

32. White House Domestic Policy Council, *Health Security*, pp. 62–63.

33. Created in 1982 to review quality and utilization in the medicare program, PROs are private nonprofit entities set in place on a state-by-state basis through competitively awarded federal contracts. Thirty-five states contract with the PROs to review quality and utilization in the medicaid program. The Health Care Financing Administration provided this information.

34. *President Clinton's Health Care Reform Proposal*, pp. 103, 451–52.

35. Ibid., p. 453.

36. *Health Security Act*, S. 1757, 103 Cong. 1 sess., p. 32.

37. Jill Zuckman, Jeffrey L. Katz, and Thomas H. Moore, "Where the Money Goes," *Congressional Quarterly Special Report*, December 11, 1993, pp. 100–01.

38. Robert H. Brook and Kathleen N. Lohr, "Will We Need to Ration Effective Health Care?" *Issues in Science and Technology*, vol. 3 (Fall 1986), p. 72.

39. Gary Clarke, in *Implementing a Reformed Health Care System*, p. 272.

40. General Accounting Office, *Medical Malpractice: Maine's Use of Practice Guidelines to Reduce Costs*, HRD-94-8 (October 1993).

41. Gina Kolata, "Mammogram Debate Moving from Test's Merits to Its Cost," *New York Times*, December 27, 1993, p. A1; see also Christine Russell, "Mammography Reassessed; NCI Deemphasizes Test for Women in Forties," *Washington Post*, December 4, 1993, p. A1; and Dana Priest, " 'Empowered' Sen. Boxer Takes on NCI Director," *Washington Post*, March 10, 1994, p. A25.

42. GAO, *Medical Malpractice*.

43. Federal auditors have recently highlighted the great variation in definitions of appropriate care by medicare's insurance carriers. Spencer Rich, "Medicare Claim Denials Vary Widely, GAO Says," *Washington Post*, March 29, 1994, p. A11.

44. Troyen A. Brennan, "Practice Guidelines and Malpractice Litigation: Collision or Cohesion?" *Journal of Health Politics, Policy and Law*, vol. 16 (Spring 1991), p. 69.

45. OTA, *Quality of Medical Care*, pp. 231, 237–46.

46. Most of the other major reform plans propose malpractice reform and establish grievance procedures. The McDermott-Wellstone, Cooper-Breaux, and Thomas-Chafee proposals also endorse ombudsmen. *Health Reform Legislation: A Comparison of Major Proposals* (Washington: Kaiser Commission on the Future of Medicaid, January 1994).

47. *President Clinton's Health Care Reform Proposal*, p. 477.

48. Ibid., p. 476.

49. Ibid., p. 479.

50. Although the Health Security Act assigns the survey function to AHCPR, the National Center for Health Statistics possesses more capacity to take the lead.

51. Ray Sweeney, in *Implementing a Reformed Health Care System*, pp. 240–41, 271.

52. Henry J. Aaron and William B. Schwartz, *The Painful Prescription* (Brookings, 1984), p. 101.

53. Kenneth E. Thorpe argues that "narrowing the gap between GNP growth and growth in health expenditures will require limits on technological innovation" and assesses regulatory mechanisms aimed at accomplishing this task. Regulation could slow diffusion by requiring exhaustive evaluation of new technologies before their introduction into medical practice. Once introduced, regulation could seek to limit the technology to certain practice settings. Either approach would be politically contentious and difficult to implement. See Kenneth E. Thorpe, "Cost Containment and National Health Care Reform: Implementation Issues," in Charles Brecher, ed., *Implementation Issues and National Health Care Reform* (New York: Robert F. Wagner Graduate School of Public Service, 1992), pp. 90–91; see also Henry J. Aaron, *Serious and Unstable Condition: Financing America's Health Care* (Brookings, 1991), pp. 48–49; and General Accounting Office, *Medical Technology: Quality Assurance Systems and Global Markets*, PEMD-93-15 (August 1993).

54. Senators Tom Harkin and Mark Hatfield introduced legislation that would place 1 percent of all health insurance premiums in a trust fund that would go to NIH. See Hilary Stout, "Search for Cures Gets Short Shrift in Health-Care Plans," *Wall Street Journal*, April 1, 1994, pp. B1–2.

55. Lawrence D. Brown, "Political Evolution of Federal Health Care Regulation," *Health Affairs*, vol. 11 (Winter 1992), pp. 17–37.

Chapter Five

1. Commerce Clearing House, *President Clinton's Health Care Reform Proposal: Health Security Act: CCH Professional Summary and Text of Bill* (Chicago: Commerce Clearing House, 1993) (hereinafter referred to as the Health Security Act).

2. The field of medicine is divided into twenty-five specialties and fifty-seven subspecialties. Doctors who are trained in family medicine, general internal medicine, and general pediatrics are commonly considered generalists. The Clinton plan adds to this definition doctors trained in obstetrics and gynecology. Health Security Act, sec. 3012. The federal government classifies communities with inadequate supplies of health care professionals as "health manpower shortage areas." Between 1978 and 1992, the number of such commu-

nities rose by 83 percent, to 2,271. Steven A. Schroeder, "Reform and the Physician Work Force," *Domestic Affairs*, vol. 2 (Winter 1993–94), p. 118.

3. Philip R. Lee, written testimony on the Health Security Act, before the Senate Committee on Labor and Human Resources, January 26, 1994, p. 1.

4. Steven A. Schroeder and Lewis G. Sandy, "Specialty Distribution of U.S. Physicians: The Invisible Driver of Health Care Costs," *New England Journal of Medicine*, April 1, 1993, pp. 961–63.

5. Health Security Act, secs. 3064, 3001, 3012.

6. Health Security Act, sec. 3062 and Title 3, subtitles E and G.

7. Health Security Act, sec. 1329. Under the Health Security Act, health plans would compete to provide a basic benefit package to eligible consumers. Health alliances would be created to organize and supervise the competition.

8. Health Security Act, secs. 1431, 1432, 1203.

9. The Hospital Survey and Construction Act of 1946 (generally referred to as the Hill-Burton act).

10. Frank J. Thompson, *Health Policy and the Bureaucracy: Politics and Implementation* (MIT Press, 1981), p. 32.

11. The National Commission on the State and Local Public Service, *Frustrated Federalism: Rx for State and Local Health Care Reform* (Albany, N.Y.: Rockefeller Institute of Public Affairs, 1993), p. 31. To be sure, Hill-Burton is not the only explanation for the surge in hospital construction. The growth of third-party insurance, for example, which generously reimbursed hospitals for the care they rendered, contributed significantly as well.

12. At the same time, however, many Hill-Burton facilities both discriminated against minorities and reneged on their obligation to provide some free services to low-income residents. Thompson, *Health Policy and the Bureaucracy*, pp. 38–40.

13. In 1992 the bed occupancy rate for community hospitals averaged 62 percent (with the percentage in the nation's rural hospitals even lower). Prospective Payment Assessment Commission, *Medicare and the American Health Care System: Report to the Congress* (Washington, June 1993), p. 81.

14. Robert M. Politzer and others, "Primary Care Physician Supply and the Medically Underserved," *Journal of the American Medical Association*, July 3, 1991, pp. 104–09.

15. Thompson, *Health Policy and the Bureaucracy*, p. 80.

16. Barry Stimmel, "The Crisis in Primary Care and the Role of Medical Schools," *Journal of the American Medical Association*, October 21, 1992, pp. 2060–65.

17. Stephen S. Mick, "Contradictory Policies for Foreign Medical Graduates," *Health Affairs*, vol. 6 (Fall 1987), pp. 5–18.

18. Steven Jonas, "Health Manpower: With an Emphasis on Physicians," in Anthony R. Kovner, ed., *Health Care Delivery in the United States*, 4th ed. (New York: Springer, 1990), p. 69.

19. Department of Health and Human Services, *Health Personnel in the United States: Eighth Report to Congress, 1991* (Rockville, Md.: September 1992), p. 96.

20. Department of Health and Human Services, *Factbook: Health Personnel United States* (1993), table 101.

21. Thompson, *Health Policy and the Bureaucracy*, p. 81.

22. Politzer and others, "Primary Care Physician Supply and the Medically Underserved," pp. 104, 107.

23. Thompson, *Health Policy and the Bureaucracy*, p. 82.

24. Association of American Medical Colleges, *AAMC Data Book* (Washington, December 1992), table B13; and Henry A. Waxman, "Health Care Workforce Reforms: Meeting Primary Care Needs," *Academic Medicine*, vol. 68 (December 1993), pp. 898–90.

25. The Emergency Health Personnel Act of 1970.

26. General Accounting Office, *National Health Service Corps: Program Unable to Meet Need for Physicians in Underserved Areas*, HRD-90-128 (August 1990), pp. 3, 6, 14; Thompson, *Health Policy and the Bureaucracy*, p. 103; and Politzer and others, "Primary Care Physician Supply and the Medically Underserved," p. 105.

27. The Reagan official quoted is Robert Graham, acting administrator of the Human Resources Administration, Department of Health and Human Services. Lawrence S. Lewin and Robert A. Derzon, "Health Professions Education: State Responsibilities under the New Federalism," *Health Affairs*, vol. 1 (Spring 1982), p. 72.

28. Association of American Medical Colleges, *AAMC Data Book*, table E2.

29. Ibid.

30. Politzer and others, "Primary Care Physician Supply and the Medically Underserved," p. 105; Alice Sardell, "Capacity-Building for the Delivery for Transmedical Services: Recruitment and Retention of Physicians for Public Service," paper prepared for the National Commission on the State and Local Public Service (Albany, N.Y.: Rockefeller Institute of Public Affairs, 1992), pp. 12–13; and Eli Ginzberg, "Improving Health Care for the Poor: Lessons from the 1980s," *Journal of the American Medical Association*, February 9, 1994, p. 465.

31. For example, see *Temple University* v. *White*, 941 F.2d 201 (3d Cir. 1991).

32. Prospective Payment Assessment Commission, *Medicare and the American Health Care System*, p. 136; Robert Pear, "Medicare Paying Doctors 59% of Insurers' Rate, Panel Finds," *New York Times*, April 5, 1994, p. A10; and Ginzberg, "Improving Health Care for the Poor," p. 465.

33. This is an effective cost containment device: hospitals now have an economic incentive to reduce actual costs, rather than expand costs. See generally, Louise B. Russell, *Medicare's New Hospital Payment System: Is It Working?* (Brookings, 1989).

34. Ibid., p. 12; and Fitzhugh Mullan, Marc L. Rivo, and Robert M. Politzer, "Doctors, Dollars, and Determination: Making Physician Work-Force Policy, *Health Affairs*, vol. 12 (1993 supplement), p. 143.

35. Schroeder and Sandy, "Specialty Distribution of U.S. Physicians."

36. Association of American Medical Colleges, *AAMC Data Book*, table B13.

37. Jack M. Colwill, interview in *Advances*, vol. 6 (Fall 1993), p. 4.

38. Council on Graduate Medical Education, *Improving Access to Health Care through Physician Workforce Reform: Directions for the 21st Century* (Rockville, Md.: Public Health Service, 1992); Physician Payment Review Commission, "Reforming Graduate Medical Education," in *Annual Report to Congress, 1993* (Washington, 1993); Pew Health Professions Commission, *Primary Care Workforce 2000: Federal Health Policy Strategies* (San Francisco, 1993); and Josiah Macy, Jr., Foundation, *Josiah Macy, Jr., Foundation Annual Report* (New York, 1992). The Physician Payment Review Commission was the only one of the four organizations not to support a mandatory 50-50 allocation; instead it suggested that "decisions about the number of residencies per specialty should be made by a federal body

created for this purpose." Physician Payment Review Commission, "Reforming Graduate Medical Education," p. 68.

39. H.R. 2804. See generally, Waxman, "Health Care Workforce Reforms."

40. Stuart Bondurant, written testimony on the Health Security Act before the Senate Committee on Labor and Human Resources, January 26, 1994, p. 3.

41. American Medical Association, *Joint Report of the Council on Medical Education and the Council on Long Range Planning and Development on Guidelines for Physician Workforce Planning* (Chicago, 1993), p. 6.

42. Richard A. Cooper, "Educating Physicians for a Balanced Workforce in the 21st Century," paper prepared for the 1993 AMA Presidents' Forum, p. 11.

43. Association of American Medical Colleges, *AAMC Data Book*, table B13.

44. *Implementing a Reformed Health Care System: The View from the Field*, transcript of conference held at the Nelson A. Rockefeller Institute of Government, Albany, N.Y., November 1993, p. 87.

45. Cooper, "Educating Physicians for a Balanced Workforce," p. 18; and Schroeder, "Reform and the Physician Work Force," pp. 128–30.

46. Bondurant, written testimony, January 26, 1994; and Donald G. Kassebaum and Philip Szenas, "Specialty Preferences of 1993 Medical School Graduates," *Academic Medicine*, vol. 68 (November 1993), p. 867.

47. David A. Kindig, James M. Cultice, and Fitzhugh Mullan, "The Elusive Generalist Physician: Can We Reach a 50% Goal?" *Journal of the American Medical Association*, September 1, 1993, pp. 1069–73.

48. Schroeder, "Reform and the Physician Work Force," p. 121.

49. *Implementing a Reformed Health Care System*, p. 126.

50. Jack Y. Krakower, Paul Jolly, and Robert Beran, "U.S. Medical School Finances," *Journal of the American Medical Association*, September 1, 1993, p. 1085.

51. Health Security Act, sec. 3013.

52. Bondurant, written testimony, January 26, 1994, p. 24.

53. Costs at teaching hospitals are, on average, 25 percent higher than at other hospitals. Lee, written testimony, January 26, 1994, p. 7.

54. Health Security Act, sec. 3131; and Bondurant, written testimony, January 26, 1994, p. 10.

55. Health Security Act, sec. 3012; Marc L. Rivo, Debbie M. Jackson, and Lawrence Clare, "Comparing Physician Workforce Reform Recommendations," *Journal of the American Medical Association*, September 1, 1993, p. 1084; and Lee, written testimony, January 26, 1994, pp. 3, 5.

56. Jerome P. Kassirer, "Primary Care and the Affliction of Internal Medicine," *New England Journal of Medicine*, March 4, 1993, p. 649.

57. Jan Towers, written testimony on the Workforce in Health Care Reform, before the House Energy and Commerce Subcommittee on Health and the Environment, January 25, 1994, p. 2; and Ann Elderkin, written testimony on Workforce Issues, before the Senate Labor and Human Resources Committee, January 26, 1994, p. 1.

58. Schroeder, "Reform and the Physician Work Force," p. 128.

59. Ibid., p. 129.

60. Towers, written testimony, January 25, 1994, p. 1.

61. Edward H. O'Neil, written testimony on the Health Security Act, before the Senate Committee on Labor and Human Resources, January 26, 1994, p. 7.

62. Adrienne Petty, "Nurse Practitioners Fight Job Restrictions," *Wall Street Journal*, September 3, 1993, p. B1.

63. *Implementing a Reformed Health Care System*, pp. 90–91.

64. Health Security Act, sec. 1161.

65. Linda H. Aiken and others, "Contribution of Specialists to the Delivery of Primary Care," *New England Journal of Medicine*, June 14, 1979, pp. 1363–76. However, specialists typically provide a more expensive brand of primary care than do generalists.

66. The passage and subsequent repeal of the medicare catastrophic legislation is instructive. In that case, organized interests persuaded large numbers of senior citizens that legislation just enacted would cause them to pay twice for catastrophic insurance. The political opposition became so strong that Congress repealed much of the bill, even though the campaign against it was based largely on inaccurate information.

67. States supervise much of the private health insurance industry, administer the public insurance program for the poor (medicaid), regulate the quality of care delivered by many medical providers, fund (with local governments) nearly 14 percent of the nation's health care bill, and operate their own workers' compensation system, medical malpractice system, and medical education system.

68. Health Security Act, sec. 1203

69. National Commission on the State and Local Public Service, *Frustrated Federalism*, p. 46.

70. *Implementing a Reformed Health Care System*, p. 91.

71. Bondurant, written testimony, January 26, 1994, p. 24.

72. Governor's Health Care Advisory Board Task Force on the Clinton Health Care Plan, *Report to the Governor* (January 5, 1994), p. 17.

73. The effort to rank programs by quality will undoubtedly lead to ongoing litigation.

74. Jack Colwill, written testimony on the Health Security Act, before the Senate Committee on Labor and Human Resources, January 26, 1994, p. 5.

75. Philip R. Lee, written testimony on the Health Security Act, before the Subcommittee on Health and the Environment of the House Committee on Energy and Commerce, January 25, 1994, p. 3.

Chapter Six

1. See Richard P. Nathan, *Turning Promises into Performance* (Columbia University Press, 1993).

2. Donald F. Kettl, *Sharing Power: Public Governance and Private Markets* (Brookings, 1993), pp. 99–127.

3. Celia W. Dugger, "Program to Preserve Families Draws Child-Welfare Debate," *New York Times*, August 6, 1993, p. A1.

4. National Research Council, *Losing Generations: Adolescents in High-Risk Settings* (National Academy Press, 1993).

5. Douglas J. Besharov, "Fresh Start," *New Republic*, June 14, 1993, pp. 14–16; and Jeffrey L. Katz, "Head Start Funding Nears Legislative Crossroad," *Congressional Quarterly Weekly Report*, March 5, 1994, pp. 541–47.

6. Douglas J. Besharov, "Fresh Start," pp. 14–16; and James Q. Wilson, "In Loco Parentis," *Brookings Review* (Fall 1993), p. 14.

7. John J. DiIulio, Jr., Steve Smith, and Aaron Saiger, "Prisoner of Federalism: The National Government's Limited Role in Crime Control," in James Q. Wilson and Joan Petersilia, eds., *Crime and Public Policy* (Institute for Contemporary Studies, forthcoming 1994).

8. John J. DiIulio, Jr., "Crime," in Henry J. Aaron and Charles L. Schultze, eds., *Setting Domestic Priorities: What Can Government Do?* (Brookings, 1992).

9. James Q. Wilson, "Can the Bureaucracy Be Deregulated? Lessons from Government Agencies," in John J. DiIulio, Jr., ed., *Deregulating the Public Service: Can Government Be Improved?* (Brookings, 1994), pp. 42–43.

10. Wilson, "Can the Bureaucracy Be Deregulated?" p. 44; and Mark Alan Hughes, "Mass Transit Agencies: Deregulating Where the Rubber Meets the Road?" in John J. DiIulio, Jr., ed., *Deregulating the Public Service: Can Government be Improved?* (Brookings, 1994), pp. 236–48.

11. John J. DiIulio, Jr., Gerald Garvey, and Donald F. Kettl, *Improving Government Performance: An Owner's Manual* (Brookings, 1993), p. 42.

12. Martha Derthick, *New Towns In-Town: Why a Federal Program Failed* (Washington: Urban Institute, 1972).

13. Jeffrey L. Pressman and Aaron Wildavsky, *Implementation: How Great Expectations in Washington Are Dashed in Oakland; Or, Why It's Amazing that Federal Programs Work at All, This Being a Saga of the Economic Development Administration as Told by Two Sympathetic Observers Who Seek to Build Morals on a Foundation of Ruined Hopes* (University of California Press, 1979).

14. General Accounting Office, *Pollution Prevention: EPA Should Reexamine the Objectives and Sustainability of State Programs*, PEMD-94-8 (January 1994), p. 3.

15. See Kettl, *Sharing Power*.

16. See National Academy of Public Administration, *Report on Government Corporations* (Washington, August 1981); Harold Seidman, "The Quasi World of the Federal Government," *Brookings Review*, vol. 6 (Summer 1988), pp. 23–27; Harold Seidman and Robert Gilmour, *Politics, Position, and Power: From the Positive to the Regulatory State*, 4th ed. (Oxford University Press, 1986); and Thomas H. Stanton, *Government Sponsored Enterprises: Their Benefits and Costs as Instruments of Federal Policy* (Washington: Association of Reserve City Bankers, April 1988).

Chapter Seven

1. Lawrence D. Brown, "Dogmatic Slumbers: American Business and Health Policy," *Journal of Health Politics, Policy and Law*, vol. 18 (Summer 1993), pp. 339–57.

2. On the distinction see Lawrence D. Brown, "Political Evolution of Federal Health Care Regulation," *Health Affairs*, vol. 11 (Winter 1992), pp. 17–37.

3. Albert O. Hirschman, *Exit, Voice, and Loyalty: Responses to Decline in Firms, Organizations, and States* (Harvard University Press, 1970).

4. National Commission on the State and Local Public Service, *Frustrated Federalism: Rx for State and Local Health Care Reform; The Second Report* (Albany: Nelson A. Rockefeller Institute of Government, 1993).

Index